THE QUICK & EASY

AYURVEDIC COOKBOOK

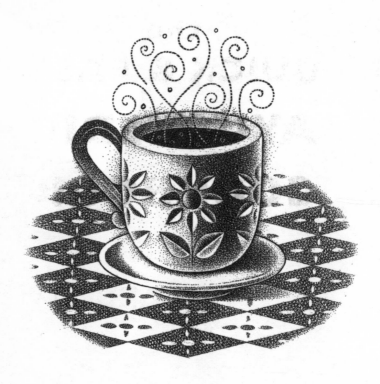

THE *QUICK & EASY*

AYURVEDIC COOKBOOK

Eileen Keavy Smith

TUTTLE PUBLISHING
Tokyo • Rutland, Vermont • Singapore

Published by Tuttle Publishing, an imprint of Periplus Editions (HK) Ltd., with editorial offices at 364 Innovation Drive, North Clarendon, Vermont 05759 U.S.A.

Copyright © 2000 Eileen Keavy Smith
Cover photo © Stewart Leishman Photography

The Library of Congress has cataloged the earlier edition as follows:

Smith, Eileen Keavy.
       The quick and easy ayurvedic cookbook / Eileen Keavy Smith.
       x, 150 p. : ill. ; 23 cm.
       Includes index.
       ISBN 1-885203-74-8 (pb)
       1. Nutrition. 2. Medicine, Ayurvedic. 3. Health. I. Title.
       RA784.S585 1999
       613.2--dc21   98-56150
                                        CIP

ISBN 978-0-8048-3906-8

Distributed by

North America, Latin America & Europe
Tuttle Publishing
364 Innovation Drive
North Clarendon, VT 05759-9436 U.S.A.
Tel: 1 (802) 773-8930; Fax: 1 (802) 773-6993
info@tuttlepublishing.com
www.tuttlepublishing.com

Japan
Tuttle Publishing
Yaekari Building, 3rd Floor
5-4-12 Osaki; Shinagawa-ku
Tokyo 141 0032
Tel: (81) 03 5437-0171; Fax: (81) 03 5437-0755
tuttle-sales@gol.com

Asia Pacific
Berkeley Books Pte. Ltd.
61 Tai Seng Avenue, #02-12
Singapore 534167
Tel: (65) 6280-1330; Fax: (65) 6280-6290
inquiries@periplus.com.sg
www.periplus.com

12 11 10 09   10 9 8 7 6 5 4 3 2

Printed in Singapore

TUTTLE PUBLISHING® is a registered trademark of Tuttle Publishing, a division of Periplus Editions (HK) Ltd.

To my loving husband, Rob, who contributed a discerning palate, a sympathetic ear and an editorial eye.

TABLE OF CONTENTS

PREFACE

Several years ago, I read a book about Ayurveda that explained very clearly why and how our health and enjoyment of life are affected by all sorts of influences. *Ayurveda* (pronounced eye-your-vay'-dah) is a Sanskrit word meaning "the science of life." The holistic Ayurvedic tradition has its roots in ancient India, and is gaining popularity in the West as we learn of its benefits. Ayurveda teaches that these influences, such as food, tastes, odors, the weather, music and other sounds, physical exercise, and much more can affect people in different ways, depending upon each person's individual constitution. For instance, I learned why I can't tolerate a blast of direct air from an air conditioner, while others find it refreshing. I learned interesting and useful things about eating and health, such as why I have problems with heartburn during the summer, but have virtually no heartburn during the rest of the year. Ayurveda goes even further by recommending how an individual can modify these influences to suit his or her own constitution. A self-test will help you determine your Ayurvedic constitution (page 8).

This cookbook is the result of having organized my meals according to Ayurvedic principles. My main objective is to keep meal planning and cooking as simple as possible. I am a busy American woman with a full-time job. I don't have time to hunt for unusual ingredients or to spend hours every day making complicated recipes from scratch. Several Ayurvedic cookbooks are listed in the Resources section of this book. All recipes in these cookbooks are vegetarian, and some of them call for ingredients that are hard to find. I enjoy using these cookbooks from time to time, but find them impractical for daily use. So, I have adapted my favorite, easily prepared recipes to fit the basic rules of Ayurvedic cooking and eating.

As you read and use this book, please keep in mind not just the Ayurvedic principles that it teaches you, but also some universal nutrition principles of which you are, most likely, already aware. The first step to practicing Ayurvedic principles is to join the increasing number of consumers who are enjoying more fresh, locally grown, organic foods. Ayurveda is all about being in tune with nature, and the movement toward eco-friendly agriculture and "green" consumerism is a hopeful sign that our society is moving in a more Ayurvedic direction. Second, try not to sacrifice your health and well-being for the sake of time-saving convenience. While it occasionally may be necessary to stop at a fast food restaurant, or use canned or frozen foods instead of fresh, try not to make this your norm. (However, when you do use canned or frozen food, use organic brands!) Third, remember to balance good nutrition with adequate physical exercise. Even when you eat healthy food, it's still possible to overeat—to take in more calories than you expend in movement—and therefore to become overweight.

The information about Ayurveda in this book is very basic. If you would like to know more about the subject, several excellent books are listed in the Resources section, along with the names, addresses and phone numbers of three Ayurvedic organizations located in the United States. I have provided a general description of what Ayurveda is, how it relates to food, and what can be eaten to help relieve some common occasional ailments. As with any ailment, if symptoms persist or worsen, a physician's opinion should be sought.

I hope that my friends and other readers will enjoy learning about Ayurveda and how to apply it to meal planning and cooking. I celebrate the unfolding of optimal health and wellness in all of us!

PART ONE

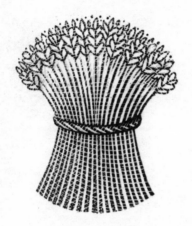

INTRODUCTION TO AYURVEDA

Ayurveda originated in India, beginning around 3000 BC. The fundamental principles of Ayurveda were discovered by ancient Rishis (Sanskrit, "seers of truth"). It was these same Rishis who developed India's original systems of Yoga and meditation. Collectively, all of these systems are known as Vedic Science. Ayurveda spread with Vedic and Hindu culture to many parts of the world and is thought to have influenced ancient Greek medicine.

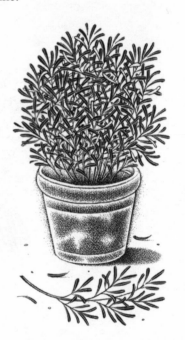

Following the discovery of its basic principles, the body of knowledge known as Ayurveda grew as practitioners of the science made very meticulous observations of human beings and the natural world. An enormous amount of information has been collected about various food, plant and mineral substances, physical activities, environmental conditions, cycles of time, and how they affect the health of human beings. This body of information was at first committed to memory and spoken in verse, and eventually was recorded in the ancient Indian language of Sanskrit. Ayurveda, as a medical science, is still practiced today in India and other parts of the Eastern world. A recent interest among Western physicians is part of a renewed inquiry into methods of preventative, holistic, cost-effective systems of health care.

THE THREE PILLARS OF LIFE

A central principle of Ayurveda encompasses three fundamental forces that regulate life. They are referred to metaphorically as air, fire and water. These three operating principles, also called the *doshas* (pronounced doe'shas), are present in all life forms, from a human being to a blade of grass. They are not physical in the sense of having tangible form, but are the very subtle energies present in all matter.

Vata (pronounced vah'-tah) is the Sanskrit word for the air principle. It is the subtle force behind all movement in the body. It is the wind that keeps things in motion, such as the transmission of messages throughout the nervous system. *Pitta,* (pronounced pit'-tah) is the Sanskrit word for the fire principle. It is the force that underlies the processes of digestion and metabolism, and the fire that burns food to fuel the body. *Kapha* (pronounced kah'-fah) is the Sanskrit word for the elemental force that upholds both density and fluidity in the body. It is the water that lubricates the body and also brings structure and stability.

The following chart lists some of the characteristics, or qualities, of each dosha. These qualities can have a healthy or unhealthy effect on our bodies and minds, depending upon the proportion of each dosha influencing our physiology at any given time. For instance, if there is too much vata in your body, symptoms associated with coldness and dryness can result. If your vata is balanced, you will not have these symptoms.

QUALITIES OF EACH DOSHA

VATA (AIR)	PITTA (FIRE)	KAPHA (WATER)
Cold	Hot	Cold
Light	Light	Heavy
Dry	Wet	Wet
Bitter	Sour	Sweet
Active	Active	Slow
Increases during cold, dry weather	*Increases during hot weather*	*Increases during cold, wet weather*

THE INDIVIDUAL CONSTITUTION

All three of the doshas must be present in a living organism. Not all organisms, however, have the same ratio of one dosha to the other two. Some organisms have more vata than they have pitta or kapha. Some have more kapha in relation to vata and pitta, and so on. Most of us have a dominant dosha that influences our physical and mental characteristics.

According to Ayurveda, we are each born with our own unique mixture of the three doshas. This is the individual's *constitution,* (*Prakruti* in Sanskrit), which is genetically determined at the time of conception. It is your constitution that determines your physical and mental characteristics such as your body frame, your ideal body weight, the color and texture of your hair and skin, and your temperament. Most of us have a dominant dosha (vata, pitta or kapha) that influences our physical and mental charateristics.

The following self-test will allow you to get a general idea of your individual constitution. Read each statement and circle a number from 0 to 4, depending upon how true each answer is for you. Circle 0 if it is not true at all. Circle 4 if it is very true. Total your score for each dosha by adding the circled numbers. Write down your total for each dosha.

The test is taken from The Healthy Family Handbook, *by Louise Taylor and Lisa Marie Nelson, and published by Tuttle Publishing.*

VATA	Not True at All				Very True
I don't like cold weather	0	1	2	3	4
I don't gain weight easily	0	1	2	3	4
I often become anxious and restless	0	1	2	3	4
My moods change quickly	0	1	2	3	4
I am creative, imaginative	0	1	2	3	4
I walk quickly	0	1	2	3	4
I have difficulty falling or staying asleep	0	1	2	3	4
I tend to make and change friends	0	1	2	3	4
I learn quickly and forget quickly	0	1	2	3	4
I become constipated easily	0	1	2	3	4
Under stress I am easily excited	0	1	2	3	4
I have an irregular appetite	0	1	2	3	4
My skin tends to be dry, rough, especially in winter	0	1	2	3	4
My feet and hands tend to be cold	0	1	2	3	4
My hair tends to be dry	0	1	2	3	4

VATA TOTAL _____

PITTA	Not True at All			Very True	
I don't like hot weather	0	1	2	3	4
My weight is average for my build	0	1	2	3	4
I tend to become intense, irritable	0	1	2	3	4
My moods are intense and change slowly	0	1	2	3	4
I am intelligent, efficient, a perfectionist	0	1	2	3	4
I have a determined walk	0	1	2	3	4
I sleep well, for an average length of time	0	1	2	3	4
Most of my friends are work-related	0	1	2	3	4
I have a good general memory	0	1	2	3	4
I have regular bowel habits	0	1	2	3	4
Under stress, I am easily angered, critical	0	1	2	3	4
I am uncomfortable skipping meals	0	1	2	3	4
My skin is soft, ruddy	0	1	2	3	4
I like cold foods and drinks	0	1	2	3	4
My hair is fine, thin, reddish, or prematurely gray	0	1	2	3	4

PITTA TOTAL _____

KAPHA	Not True at All				Very True
I don't like damp, cool weather	0	1	2	3	4
I gain weight easily	0	1	2	3	4
I can be slow or depressed	0	1	2	3	4
My moods are mostly steady	0	1	2	3	4
My mind is calm, steady, stable	0	1	2	3	4
My walk is slow and steady	0	1	2	3	4
I generally sleep long and soundly	0	1	2	3	4
My friendships are longlasting, sincere	0	1	2	3	4
I have a good longterm memory	0	1	2	3	4
I eat and digest slowly	0	1	2	3	4
I am stubborn, not easily ruffled	0	1	2	3	4
I can skip meals easily	0	1	2	3	4
My skin is oily, moist	0	1	2	3	4
I have good stamina, steady energy level	0	1	2	3	4

KAPHA TOTAL _____

COMPARATIVE TOTALS

VATA＿＿＿＿＿＿＿

PITTA＿＿＿＿＿＿

KAPHA＿＿＿＿＿＿

Your highest-scoring dosha is your dominant dosha. For example, if you scored 42 for vata, 30 for pitta and 21 for kapha, your individual constitution is vata. Many people have two high-scoring doshas, which means both doshas dominate. I score lowest for vata and score nearly the same for pitta and kapha, with kapha a few points ahead of pitta. My constitution, therefore, is kapha-pitta. In my constitution, kapha leads, but not by much. If all three doshas have about the same score, you are tri-doshic. *This is rare, however.*

BALANCE AND IMBALANCE

Ayurveda teaches that a perfect balance will maintain the same proportion of the three doshas with which you were born. Your inborn constitution represents your balanced state of health. If your present ratio of doshas does not match your constitution, you are out of balance and are likely to be experiencing some degree of poor health.

Most of us recognize when we are in good health. During daily activities we feel alert, energetic and physically comfortable. We get enough deep sleep and wake up refreshed. When there is a lack of energy, physical discomfort, irritability or sleeplessness, something is "out of whack." This something is likely to be one (or more) of the doshas.

What causes the imbalance? Ayurveda suggests that, by the principle of resonance, like increases like. A hot summer day will increase pitta (fire) in the body. By the same token, a cold day will decrease pitta. Since kapha (water) is cold and wet, a cold and rainy day will increase kapha. Environmental conditions influence the balance of the doshas and come in the form of climate, food, odors, noises or any outside influence on the body. Emotional states are also considered environmental conditions. The emotion of anger, for instance, will elevate pitta, the fire principle.

To illustrate how environmental conditions can upset the balance of the doshas, I'll use two examples from my own situation. I can't tolerate direct air from an air conditioner. My constitution is kapha-pitta. Since one of the qualities of kapha is coldness, I tend to become cold easily. The warming quality of pitta moderates this tendency somewhat, but not enough to eliminate it. Direct flow from an air conditioner throws me out of balance and can result in sinus congestion and sneezing, which are typical signs of a kapha imbalance. Low, indirect air conditioning or a slow-running fan work just fine in my case.

Another example concerns a pitta imbalance that occurs in the summertime. I love spicy food and have no problem digesting it most of the year. But in the summer, spicy food gives me heartburn. So, I avoid spicy food and instead, eat foods that are cooling. No more heartburn!

The following chart lists the common symptoms that result when each of the doshas is elevated to the point of causing an imbalance in the body.

COMMON SYMPTOMS OF IMBALANCE

This chart lists the symptoms most commonly associated with an imbalance in each of the doshas, not every possible symptom.

VATA	PITTA	KAPHA
Dry skin	Skin inflammation	Oily, sticky skin
Constipation	Heartburn	Slow, heavy digestion
Intestinal gas	Acid indigestion	Lethargy
Anxiety	Diarrhea	Depression
Insomnia	Hot flashes	Sinus congestion
Aching pain	Excess sweating	Common cold
Poor circulation	Bloodshot eyes	Heavy sleep
Weight loss	Anger, hostility	Weight gain

AYURVEDA AND FOOD

According to Ayurveda, all life is regulated by the three doshas. Our food comes from living organisms, so food, like our bodies, also has the three doshas within it. Like us, each kind of food has its own combination of air, fire and water. For example, bananas, being sweet, wet and sticky, have the qualities of kapha.

Since bananas have a high proportion of kapha, eating one is likely to elevate your own level of kapha. So, if you have sinus congestion (a typical symptom of having too much kapha), eating a banana may worsen the condition. Eating an apple, however, would be a good idea. Apples have an astringent (drying) quality, a characteristic of vata (air). The apple might help to alleviate your sinus condition because its drying quality would reduce the mucus and congestion.

Eating foods that have qualities opposite to the dosha that is out of balance can help eventually balance the dosha and clear up the symptoms. The beneficial results of eating foods that balance a particular dosha will probably be gradual, taking a few hours or even days, depending upon the extensiveness of the imbalance. A sniffle, for instance, may clear up in a few hours after eating a spicy, kapha-balancing meal. The alleviation of an advanced case of sinus congestion, however, may require a week or more of kapha-balancing meals.

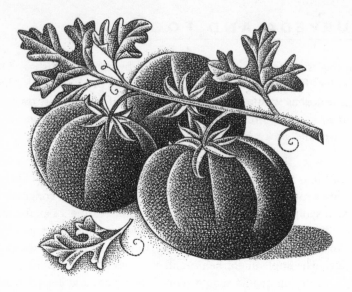

During the 5000 years of Ayurveda's development, all types of foods have been analyzed for their affect on the balance of our doshas. It has been found that the way a food influences our doshas is largely a matter of its taste. Ayurveda categorizes tastes into the following six types:

- Sweet (bread, honey and milk)
- Sour (vinegar, grapefruit)
- Salty (table salt, soy sauce)
- Bitter (black coffee, mustard greens)
- Pungent (hot spices, garlic)
- Astringent (dry and mealy, as in lima beans and apples)

Vata (air) is elevated by foods that taste bitter, pungent or astringent. Vata is lowered by foods that taste sweet, sour or salty.

Pitta (fire) is elevated by foods that taste sour, salty or pungent. Pitta is lowered by foods that taste sweet, bitter or astringent.

Kapha (water) is elevated by foods that taste sweet, sour or salty. Kapha is lowered by foods that taste bitter, pungent or astringent.

To maintain balanced doshas and therefore health, Ayurveda recommends including at least a little of all six tastes in your daily food intake. In order to include all six tastes, you must eat from a wide variety of foods, thus ensuring that you will be eating a varied and well-balanced diet. Even if you are trying to bring one of the doshas back into balance by eating foods with tastes that balance that dosha, you should still try to include the other tastes in your daily meals.

Besides taste, there are other qualities that should be considered when choosing what to eat. Lightness, heaviness, wetness, dryness and temperature are some of these other qualities. Choose foods that have qualities least like the qualities of the dosha you are trying to balance. For instance, ice cream is sweet, cold and wet. Since kapha dosha has these same three qualities, eating ice cream to balance kapha would not work. However, eating spinach, which is light, bitter and essentially dry, would help balance the kapha.

*It is not only what we eat that affects the doshas, but also how,
when and where we eat. The following is a list of poor eating habits
that can affect our doshic balance.*

- Eating at irregular intervals. According to Ayurveda, the body
  loves regular schedules. Eating your meals at consistent times every
  day is best.

- Eating too much of anything.

- Not eating enough or going on a starvation diet.

- Constantly favoring one or two tastes to the exclusion of others.
  Many people prefer sweet and salty foods and therefore don't eat a
  balanced diet. Junk foods and fast foods are predominantly sweet
  and salty.

- Eating foods that increase the effects of weather conditions. For
  example, eating a spicy Mexican meal on a hot summer day.

- Eating any of the following foods too often: red meat, fried foods,
  alcoholic beverages and foods made with lots of refined sugar.
  These foods should be eaten very seldom (if at all) since they easily
  throw the doshas out of balance.

- Eating hurriedly, in an unsettled environment, or while watching
  television, reading or listening to loud music.

Part Two of this book is a guide to the types of foods to increase or reduce, alleviating symptoms of imbalance for each dosha. Recipes are offered that emphasize foods and cooking methods that help balance each dosha. But this section need only be used when there is an imbalance, and not all the time. The basic rule of eating according to Ayurveda is that when you feel healthy and energetic, have good digestion and no pain, eat whatever healthful foods you prefer as long as you continue to feel healthy.

An excellent general guide to follow for healthy eating is the United States Department of Agriculture's Food Guide Pyramid scheme. Introduced in 1992, and later revised in 2005, the USDA Food Guide Pyramid replaced the "4 Food Group" pie chart that had been used for decades for educating the public about nutrition. Both the original Food Guide Pyramid and the 2005 revision, called MyPyramid, are shown on pages 20 and 21. The Pyramid scheme emphasizes the consumption of grains, vegetables and fruits and recommends that these foods make up the bulk of the daily diet. Smaller amounts of dairy and protein foods, according to the scheme, should make up the rest of daily food consumption, with sparse amounts of fats, oils and sweeteners rounding out the diet. This dietary scheme is perfectly acceptable to the Ayurvedic viewpoint. Ayurveda puts more emphasis on food that is derived from plant sources, and less on food derived from animal sources.

Both versions of the USDA Pyramid scheme can be useful tools when you are trying to correct a dosha imbalance. Part Two of this book contains a chapter devoted to each dosha. Each of these chapters includes a modified version of the 1992 Food Guide Pyramid with specific dosha-balancing foods listed within each food block.

The 2005 revision is still a pyramid shape, but the food blocks are now turned on their side—lined up from left to right instead of bottom to top. A human figure is shown climbing the side steps of the pyramid, promoting the importance of exercise. Fitting right in with Ayurvedic principles, it is more personalized and based on the premise that "One size does not fit all." You can explore the new pyramid by visiting the interactive website: http://www.mypyramid.gov.

Now that you have seen how Ayurvedic principles relate to food, you are ready to move on to Part Two, which will show you how to put these principles into practice.

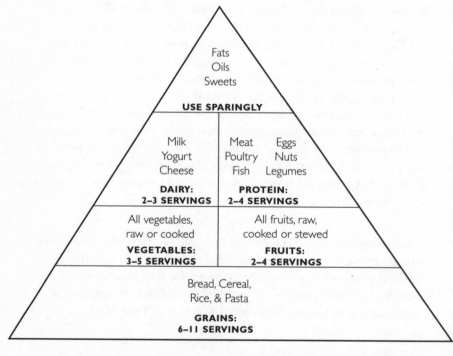

Fats
Oils
Sweets

USE SPARINGLY

Milk
Yogurt
Cheese

**DAIRY:
2–3 SERVINGS**

Meat   Eggs
Poultry Nuts
Fish   Legumes

**PROTEIN:
2–4 SERVINGS**

All vegetables,
raw or cooked

**VEGETABLES:
3–5 SERVINGS**

All fruits, raw,
cooked or stewed

**FRUITS:
2–4 SERVINGS**

Bread, Cereal,
Rice, & Pasta

**GRAINS:
6–11 SERVINGS**

THE 1992 USDA FOOD GUIDE PYRAMID

MyPyramid.gov
STEPS TO A HEALTHIER YOU

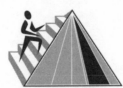

Milk Group
MyPyramid.gov

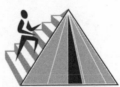

Fruit Group
MyPyramid.gov

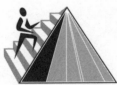

Grain Group
MyPyramid.gov

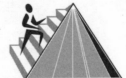

Meat & Bean Group
MyPyramid.gov

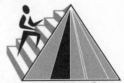

Vegetable Group
MyPyramid.gov

The 2005 USDA food good pyramid called "MyPyramid." Though I've added labels in this book to identify each food group, the official 2005 pyramid uses color-coding instead of text to identify the five major food groups. To see the full-color version of the MyPyramid scheme, and to experience its interactive components, visit http://www.Mypyramid.gov.

PART TWO

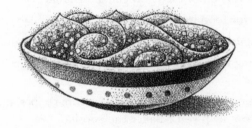

RECIPES AND GUIDELINES FOR BALANCING THE DOSHAS

The first chapter of Part Two provides background information you will need before using the recipes. The remainder of Part Two contains chapters devoted to the three doshas that include the following:

- A list of common symptoms associated with an imbalance of the dosha
- A list of foods to increase in the diet
- A list of foods to decrease in the diet
- A modified version of the Food Guide Pyramid
- Guidelines for food preparation
- Ideas for appropriate snacks, beverages, breakfasts and desserts
- Recipes using dosha-balancing ingredients and suggestions for side dishes
- An opportunity to write down your favorite recipes and other foods that can help you balance each dosha

INTRODUCTION TO THE RECIPES

WHEN TO USE THE RECIPES

Use the recipes and suggestions in this guidebook when you are experiencing one or more symptoms characteristic of a dosha imbalance. You may find this simple modification to your normal diet to be an easy and natural way to feel better. However, if your symptoms are excessive or if they persist, please get medical attention. This guidebook is not meant to provide a cure-all. A common dosha imbalance is one thing, but a serious illness is quite another.

ABOUT THE RECIPES

Unless otherwise noted, each recipe serves four adults who have moderate appetites. All ingredients can be found in most supermarkets. To make a full meal, I recommend making the side dishes that follow many of the recipes. These are items that, in my experience, complement the main dish and can help balance the dosha.

After reading about each dosha and the kinds of foods that help balance them, you will undoubtedly think of your favorite recipes and foods that will also help balance each dosha. At the end of each recipe section, space is provided for you to list your favorite main dishes, desserts, snacks, beverages and breakfasts. Over time, as you try the recipes and suggestions, more foods will come to mind that you may want to add to these lists.

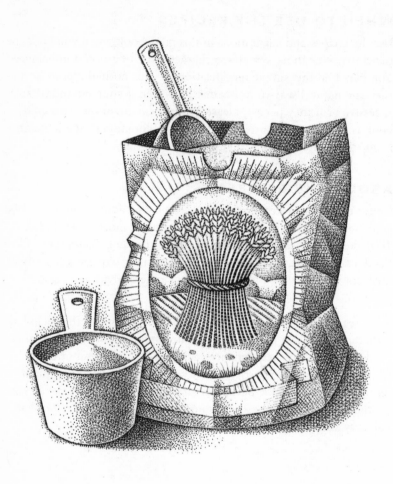

BASIC INGREDIENTS

DAIRY FOODS

Milk, cheese, creamy sauces, ice cream—most of us grew up adoring these satisfying, tasty, nutritious foods. According to Ayurveda, dairy foods very effectively balance two of the doshas, vata and pitta. Even so, Ayurveda warns that dairy foods should not be eaten in combination with meat. This is because animal protein, in general, is heavy and slow to digest. Combining two different kinds of animal protein in one meal (for example, crabmeat in a cheese sauce) can put a strain on your digestion.

There is one other warning about dairy foods. At least 15 percent of the United States population are lactose intolerant, which means they lack the enzyme lactase that allows for proper digestion of the milk sugar lactose. In these people, the undigested milk sugar passes into the large intestine where it ferments, causing bloating, painful gas and sometimes diarrhea or constipation. According to Ayurveda, lactose intolerance can be either genetically inherited or can indicate a dosha imbalance. An Ayurvedic physician may be able to prescribe treatment to cure the condition if its cause is a dosha imbalance. In any case, if you think you may be lactose intolerant, ask your physician about over-the-counter lactase tablets or liquids that can aid in the digestion of milk products.

Of course, if you are lactose intolerant or allergic, you may wish to avoid dairy products entirely. If you experience frequent kapha imbalances, avoiding them is not a bad idea. If you do not eat dairy products, however, be sure to eat plenty of green, leafy vegetables and other foods that are high in calcium. Consider taking daily calcium supplements as well.

BEANS

Beans (also called legumes) have an astringent (drying) quality and therefore are very effective for balancing kapha, the water dosha. They are also good for balancing pitta, the fire dosha, as long as they are not prepared with a lot of hot spices. The combination of beans and grains (particularly whole grains) provides excellent protein and can be effectively substituted for the protein in meat.

For many people, beans can cause intestinal gas. If vata, the air dosha, is already elevated, beans will almost certainly cause gas. Beans should be avoided if vata is out of balance.

In the recipes that call for beans, canned or dried beans can be used. Dried beans are not cooked, and therefore will have to be cooked before they can be used. Canned foods and other precooked convenience foods are generally not recommended by Ayurveda, but I feel that there are times when busy people must resort to using them. Most canned beans have added salt, and since salt tends to increase pitta and kapha, it's best to use dried beans and cook them yourself. If you prefer to use the more convenient canned beans, do not add any salt to the recipe.

All uncooked beans, except for split peas and lentils, need to be soaked for several hours (preferably overnight) before cooking. The following is a general method for cooking one cup of dried beans, which yields about three cups of cooked beans:

Place one cup of dried beans in a deep bowl and cover them with water. The water should be at least one inch above the level of the beans. Let this stand for a few minutes. Remove any debris that floats to the top of the water. Place the beans in a colander and let the water drain off.

Rinse the beans thoroughly while they're in the colander. Then place the beans in a large bowl. Pour three cups of fresh water over the beans and let them soak in the water for at least five hours or overnight. Drain the beans and place them in a large saucepan or soup pot with six cups of fresh water. To help reduce the possibility of intestinal gas, add a generous pinch of ginger powder, curry powder or turmeric powder. Simmer, uncovered, for two to three hours, until the beans are tender.

COOKING OILS

Cooking oils, like all other foods, have their own doshic qualities. Some oils have a heating effect, some are cooling, some are heavy and some are light. Although all vegetable oils will reduce vata, I've chosen olive oil to recommend in the vata-balancing recipes. For reducing pitta, the light, sweet oils are best. I've chosen canola oil to balance pitta, although sunflower or olive oil can also be used. Canola oil and corn oil are light and have a drying quality, and so are good for balancing kapha. I've used canola in the kapha recipes, but you may substitute corn oil.

Butter is recommended rather than margarine. This is because, according to Ayurveda, margarine is more difficult to digest. Besides, as most everyone agrees, butter has better flavor. Butter balances vata, but elevates both pitta and kapha.

Actually, Ayurveda recommends *ghee* as the superior cooking oil for most recipes because, when used in moderation, it has a balancing effect on all three doshas. In the West, ghee is known as clarified butter, or butter minus the milk solids, and it is commonly used in French cuisine. There are other good reasons for using ghee. Unlike butter and other oils, it does not burn easily. And, properly prepared, it will keep for a long time in the refrigerator. Ghee can be found in most health food stores and in the international foods section of some supermarkets. But why buy it when it is so easy to make at home? Here are two methods for making about two cups of ghee:

METHOD #1 FOR MAKING GHEE

Melt a pound of *unsalted* butter in a heavy saucepan over medium heat. When it begins to froth, turn the heat to low and simmer for about an hour. Skim off the froth occasionally. The milk solids will eventually sink to the bottom of the pan, leaving a clear, golden liquid on top. Carefully pour the liquid into a jar through a piece of cheesecloth or a coffee filter. The filter will prevent the milk solids from getting into the jar. Seal the jar and store the ghee in the refrigerator. Discard the milk solids.

METHOD #2 FOR MAKING GHEE

Heat the oven to 225°F (105°C). Put a pound of *unsalted* butter in a glass baking dish or a large, glass, heat-tolerant measuring cup. Put it in the oven for about an hour, until the milk solids have settled on the bottom and a clear, golden liquid is on top. Pour the liquid into a jar through a piece of cheesecloth or a coffee filter. The filter is to prevent the milk solids from getting into the jar. Seal the jar and store the ghee in the refrigerator. Discard the milk solids.

MISSING INGREDIENTS

RED MEAT

Red meat is not included in these recipes. Even though Ayurveda does not completely prohibit the use of red meat, it cautions that it is very taxing on the digestive system and tends to throw the doshas out of balance. There are some conditions, such as severe anemia, for which Ayurvedic physicians might prescribe eating red meat. Actually, the ideal Ayurvedic diet includes no meat at all. I have chosen to include some poultry and seafood recipes in this book because they are available and practical sources of protein and, when eaten in moderation, they can have a balancing effect.

HONEY (COOKED)

Honey is an ingredient that will not be found in recipes that call for heating. Ayurvedic medicine uses honey quite liberally in its medicinal preparations and loudly sings its praises. According to Ayurveda, however, honey should never be cooked. Because honey is extremely high in pitta and so naturally very hot, the additional heat resulting from cooking can be too much for the body to balance. Adding honey to a cup of hot (not boiling) tea is acceptable, or in a salad dressing, because the honey will not be cooked.

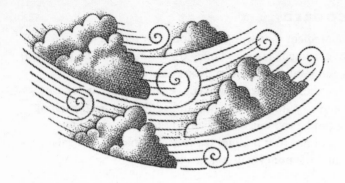

BALANCING VATA

Vata is the *air* principle. It is the wind that keeps life processes in motion, as in the transmission of messages throughout the nervous system. Its basic qualities include being very active, cold in temperature, light in weight, dry and brittle to the touch, and bitter-tasting.

"Blow winds,

and crack

your cheeks!"

Shakespeare,
King Lear

SYMPTOMS OF A VATA IMBALANCE

A vata imbalance is like a wild, windy day. There is a lot of movement going on, a lot of things being blown around. There is also a dryness, like when your lips become chapped by dry, cold air. You may have a vata imbalance if you have been experiencing one or more of the following symptoms for more than just a few days:

• Excessively dry or chapped skin
• Constipation or intestinal gas
• Unwarranted and excessive anxiety, fear or worry
• Insomnia, very light sleep or nightmares
• Muscle spasms, cramps, backache, earache or joint pains
• Poor circulation indicated by cold hands and feet
• Erratic, light appetite and consequent weight loss

POSSIBLE CAUSES

Maybe it's autumn, when leaves turn dry and crumble underfoot. Or perhaps the cold, dry winds of early winter have begun. Late fall and early winter provide a typical vata-increasing environment.

The weather may not be affecting you; you can suffer from a vata imbalance any time of the year. Have you been eating a large quantity of dry or raw foods lately? Are you overworked, nervous or worried? Perhaps your constitution is such that you naturally have a high proportion of vata, causing you to be more vulnerable to vata imbalances.

WHAT TO EAT

If you want to reduce the symptoms of a vata imbalance, you're in luck! Typical Americans love vata-balancing foods, which tend to be sweeter, saltier and richer than foods that balance the other two doshas. Flavors to increase are sweet, salty and sour. Flavors to reduce are bitter, pungent and astringent.

Emphasizing sweet flavors does not mean eating a whole box of cookies all at once. Actually, foods like milk, bread and fruit are what Ayurveda considers sweet. Likewise, increasing salty flavors does not mean you can now pour salt all over your vegetables or popcorn. Remember, the goal should still be to get all six tastes (sweet, sour, salty, bitter, pungent and astringent) into your daily meals. To balance vata, eat more of the foods that taste sweet, salty or sour and less of the foods with the other three flavors.

FOODS TO INCREASE (+) WHEN BALANCING VATA

+ Sweet foods (bread, milk and bananas)
+ Salty foods (soy sauce)
+ Sour foods (vinegar, citrus fruit)
+ Warm, cooked foods
+ Fresh fruits (apples should be cooked; raw apples can increase vata)
+ Cooked vegetables (go easy on bitter vegetables such as mustard greens and turnip greens)
+ Wheat and other grains, baked goods
+ Chicken and turkey
+ Eggs
+ Seafood (any kind)
+ Dairy foods
+ Nuts (any kind)

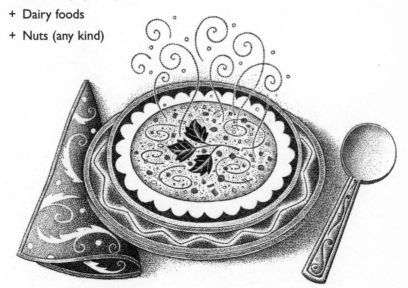

FOODS TO REDUCE (-) WHEN BALANCING VATA

- Bitter foods (black coffee, mustard greens)
- Pungent foods (hot peppers, cumin)
- Astringent foods (lima beans, raw apples)
- Cold foods
- Dried fruits
- Raw vegetables
- Legumes (beans, peas and lentils)
- Dry foods (crackers, chips)
- Foods containing caffeine (tea, coffee and chocolate)

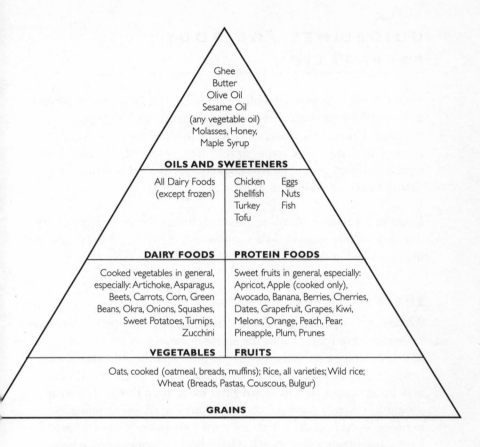

VATA-PACIFYING PYRAMID OF FOODS

A modified version of the 1992 United States Department of Agriculture's Food Guide Pyramid showing foods that help to balance vata dosha.

GUIDELINES FOR FOOD
PREPARATION

Since dryness is associated with a vata imbalance, it is very important to use cooking methods that promote moisture, such as boiling, steaming, baking in a sauce, or sautéing in ghee, butter or oil. Remember that you are trying to rehydrate your body. To ease digestion, ingredients should be well cooked and, as a general rule, food should be served warm and moist.

Good vata-balancing meals include rich Italian dishes, hearty poultry dishes, warming seafood dishes, soups and casseroles. A meal consisting of cooked grain and well-cooked vegetables is excellent.

SNACKS

According to Ayurveda, the stomach should be empty before consuming a meal. For most people, the stomach empties in about four hours, depending upon the size of the meal and the individual's metabolic rate. The erratic digestion of a person with a vata constitution may bring hunger on a more irregular basis. Even though full meals should be taken at regular intervals, a small snack may sometimes be in order. Sweet, ripe fruit makes a great vata-balancing snack, perhaps a banana or a juicy peach. Other healthy snacks include bread and cheese, a handful of nuts or a cup of yogurt.

BEVERAGES

It is very important to drink plenty of liquids when balancing vata, and warm drinks are especially beneficial. Hot apple cider is a good vata-balancer. Hot herbal teas are perfect, especially those made with ginger, cinnamon, chamomile, lemon grass, orange peel, licorice root, sarsaparilla or sassafras.

To make ginger tea:

In a saucepan, combine 1 cup (250 ml) of water with a ½-inch (1.25-cm) slice of fresh ginger (or ⅛ teaspoon of powdered ginger). Heat this mixture until it just begins to boil. Remove it from the heat and stir in a teaspoon or two of honey.

Avoid all caffeinated drinks, including tea, coffee and chocolate, as caffeine will overstimulate vata. Decaffeinated drinks are acceptable in small amounts. Avoid ice-cold drinks. Cool, not cold, fruit juices are fine.

BREAKFAST

For breakfast think warm, moist and nourishing. Hot cereals such as oatmeal, Cream of Wheat and Wheatena are wonderful for balancing vata. Serve them with milk, brown sugar and fruit. Pancakes, waffles and French toast are great, especially with a warm fruit topping. Eggs, cooked any style, are fine. Scrambled tofu can be substituted for eggs. Hot soup and a slice of bread or toast makes an excellent vata-balancing breakfast.

DESSERTS

Think of rich, sweet desserts like warm fruit cobblers and pies, rice pudding and tapioca. Christmas plum pudding really fits the bill! Desserts that warm the belly and soothe the mind are the best for balancing vata. Eat these rich desserts in moderation—an overdose could bring on a kapha imbalance. The following recipe is one of my winter favorites. It serves about 12 people.

Ginger Cake

2¹/4 cups (310 g) all-purpose flour
³/4 cup (150 g) firmly packed brown sugar
1 teaspoon baking powder
¹/2 teaspoon salt
¹/2 teaspoon baking soda
2 teaspoons powdered cinnamon
1¹/2 teaspoons powdered ginger
¹/2 teaspoon nutmeg
¹/4 teaspoon powdered cloves
³/4 cup (185 ml) molasses
³/4 cup (185 ml) canola oil
³/4 cup (185 ml) water
2 eggs

Preheat the oven to 350°F (175°C). Grease an 8 x 12-inch (20 x 30-cm) baking pan or two 4 x 8-inch (10 x 20-cm) loaf pans. Combine all of the ingredients in a large bowl. Mix with an electric mixer on low speed until just blended, then mix on medium speed for 3 minutes. Pour the mixture into the greased pan(s). Bake for 35 to 40 minutes.

Icing

1 cup (200 g) firmly packed brown sugar
1/2 cup (110 g) ghee or butter, melted
1/3 cup (80 ml) water

Mix together the sugar, ghee or butter, and water. Spread the icing evenly over the warm cake.

This cake is great served with slices of fresh fruit such as orange, peach or pear.

OTHER VATA-BALANCING DESSERT IDEAS:

- Pumpkin pie and other traditional Thanksgiving desserts
- Plum pudding and other Christmas desserts
- Pineapple upside-down cake
- Baklava (Greek pastry made with filo dough, nuts and honey)

VATA RECIPES

SEAFOOD

GRAINS

SIDE DISHES

Vegetable Burritos, Vata Style

This colorful, tasty recipe is a family favorite! The sweet flavors of the cooked vegetables combine with the somewhat sour flavor of the cheddar cheese to create an excellent vata-balancing dish. The touch of spicy salsa is not enough to negate the balancing effect, and adds variety to the overall flavor. Serve with Corn on the Cob (page 47).

4 tablespoons ghee or olive oil
I pound (500 g) summer squash or zucchini, chopped
I pound (500 g) broccoli, chopped
1/2 cup (75 g) chopped onion
2 medium tomatoes, chopped
1/4 teaspoon salt
1/4 teaspoon turmeric powder
1/8 teaspoon chili powder
4 flour tortillas (about 8 in/20 cm in diameter)
8 ounces (250 g) sharp cheddar cheese, grated
4 tablespoons mild salsa

To prepare the filling: Heat the ghee or oil in a large frying pan or skillet over medium heat. Add the squash, broccoli and onion. Sauté over medium heat for about 5 minutes. Add the tomatoes, salt, turmeric and chili powder. Stir the mixture and turn the heat to low.

To make the burritos: Heat the oven to 200°F (95°C). Melt 1/4 teaspoon ghee or butter in a small frying pan over medium heat. Place one tortilla in the pan, then sprinkle 1/2 cup (50 g) cheese evenly over the tortilla. Heat the tortilla over medium-low heat until the cheese melts. Remove the tortilla to a heat-proof plate and spoon 1/4 of the vegetable mixture onto half of the tortilla. Drizzle 1 tablespoon of salsa over the vegetables and fold the empty half of the tortilla over the full half. Keep the prepared burritos warm in the oven until all are ready to serve.

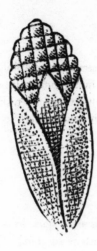

Corn on the Cob

4 ears of corn

Remove the husks and silky threads from the ears of corn. Drop the corn into a pot of boiling water. Cover the pot and let the water return to a boil. Turn off the heat and keep the pot covered. Remove the corn after about 5 minutes. Serve with butter and salt.

Shepherd's Pie

This version of Shepherd's Pie consists of chopped, steamed vegetables topped with a layer of mashed potatoes and baked. The flavor can be varied by using different vegetables, or different liquids to moisten the vegetables. Serve with whole wheat rolls and a small tossed salad.

4 medium potatoes (white potatoes or sweet potatoes)
¹/₄ cup (65 ml) milk
I tablespoon ghee or butter
¹/₄ teaspoon salt
2 pounds (I kg) assorted vegetables, chopped (such as asparagus, broccoli, carrots, celery, onion, green beans, summer squash or zucchini)
¹/₂ cup (125 ml) liquid for moistening (use chicken broth, milk or a half-and-half mixture of soy sauce and water)
4 ounces (100 g) cheddar or Parmesan cheese, grated

To make the mashed potatoes: Wash and peel the potatoes and cut them into chunks. Boil them until tender (about 10 minutes). Drain them, and mash them well. Stir in the milk, ghee or butter, and salt. Mash them again or use an electric mixer until they are smooth. Set them aside.

Preheat the oven to 400°F (200°C). Steam the chopped vegetables in two cups of water for about 5 minutes, until they are tender-crisp. Drain the vegetables and place them in a buttered 12 x 8-inch (30 x 20-cm) baking pan or in a 2-quart (2-liter) casserole dish. Add a little salt and pepper to taste. Pour the moistening liquid evenly over the vegetables. Spread the mashed potatoes in a smooth layer over the vegetables. Sprinkle the cheese evenly over the mashed potatoes. Bake the pie for about 20 minutes.

Pasta with Pesto Sauce

This is a basic recipe for pesto sauce. The main ingredients of this sauce—basil, nuts and oil—are very effective for reducing vata. This tasty, warm and filling meal should make you feel very mellow. Serve with Steamed Asparagus (page 50).

1 cup (40 g) fresh basil leaves
1/2 cup (60 g) pine nuts, walnuts or raw cashews
1 large clove garlic, peeled
2/3 cup (160 ml) olive oil
3/4 cup (75 g) grated Parmesan cheese
1 pound (500 g) pasta (preferably angel hair or linguini), cooked and
   drained

Put the basil leaves, nuts and garlic in a food processor or blender. Process until they are finely chopped, then slowly drizzle in the oil while the machine is still running. Add the cheese and briefly process until the mixture is smooth. If the sauce is too thick, add 1 tablespoon of water. Place the cooked, warm pasta in a bowl. Add the sauce to the pasta and toss with a fork until the pasta is coated.

VARIATION: *Garnish with some chopped sun-dried tomatoes that have been softened in hot water.*

Steamed Asparagus

24 asparagus

Wash the asparagus and cut off the tough bottom of each stalk. In a large saucepan, bring about 1½ cups (375 ml) of water to a boil. Place the asparagus in the boiling water, cover the pan and steam for about 5 minutes over medium heat. Drain the asparagus and serve them with melted butter or ghee.

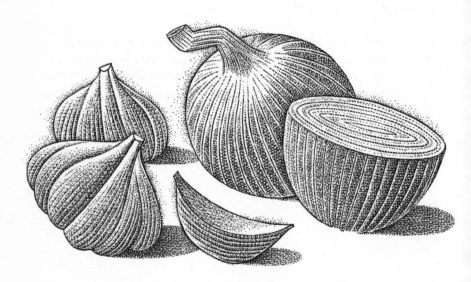

Pasta with Sweet Pepper Sauce

Surprise your taste buds with this sweet and delicate sauce for pasta, a welcome departure from traditional tomato sauce. Serve with French bread and butter.

2 red bell peppers
2 cloves garlic, peeled
3 tablespoons olive oil
1 tablespoon wine vinegar
3 tablespoons pine nuts
2 medium tomatoes, chopped, or 1 cup (240 g) canned tomatoes, chopped
1/4 teaspoon ground cinnamon
1/4 teaspoon salt
**1 pound (500 g) pasta (preferably angel hair or linguini), cooked and
  drained**

Heat the oven to 400°F (200°C). Place the whole peppers and garlic cloves on a baking sheet. Roast them for about 10 minutes. Place the peppers in cold water to loosen the skins, and then peel them.

In a blender or food processor, combine the peeled peppers, garlic, oil, vinegar, nuts, tomatoes, cinnamon and salt. Puree the mixture until it has a smooth consistency. Serve the sauce over the cooked pasta.

Creamy Butternut Soup

Cream of vegetable soups are great for balancing vata. This one makes a good accompaniment to main-dish vegetarian recipes, or it can be served by itself with any kind of bread. It goes very well with Artichoke and Spinach Casserole (page 53).

3 cups (750 ml) broth (chicken or vegetable)
1/2 teaspoon peeled and minced fresh ginger
1/2 cup (75 g) minced onion
1/2 cup (50 g) chopped celery
1 clove garlic, minced
2 cups (275 g) peeled and cubed butternut squash
1/3 cup (75 g) plain yogurt
3 tablespoons heavy cream
2 tablespoons sherry or white wine
Salt and freshly ground black pepper, to taste

In a large saucepan or soup kettle, heat 1/2 cup (125 ml) of the broth. Add the ginger, onion, celery and garlic. Cook over medium heat for 2 minutes. Add the squash and the remaining broth and cover the pan. Cook over medium-low heat for 45 minutes, or until the squash is tender. Mash the squash with a potato masher until the soup is smooth (or puree in a blender). Stir in the yogurt, cream, sherry or wine, and salt and pepper. Heat and serve.

Artichoke and Spinach Casserole

Spinach is not normally a vata-balancing vegetable, but combined with these warm and rich ingredients, it becomes perfectly appropriate and totally delicious. Serve with toasted bagels.

1 pound (500 g) spinach, rinsed and trimmed
8 ounces (250 g) cream cheese, softened
1 cup (100 g) grated Parmesan cheese
3/4 cup (185 ml) milk
1 egg, beaten
8 fresh or frozen artichoke hearts, cooked (or 8 canned artichoke hearts)
1 cup (90 g) breadcrumbs

Preheat the oven to 350°F (175°C). Put the spinach in a large bowl. In a small bowl, combine the cream cheese, 1/2 cup (50 g) of the Parmesan cheese, and the milk and egg. Mix well. Pour this mixture over the spinach and stir. Place the spinach mixture in a baking dish. Arrange the cooked artichoke hearts on top. Sprinkle with breadcrumbs and the remaining Parmesan cheese. Bake for 30 minutes.

Green Bean Stir-Fry with Nuts

Oriental stir-fry is a great choice for balancing vata. The flavors are basically sweet and salty. Many varieties of vegetables can be used. Nuts add protein as well as a crunchy texture. Serve with steamed rice.

1 pound (500 g) fresh green beans, rinsed and cut into 1-inch (2.5 cm) pieces
3 tablespoons canola or peanut oil
1 small onion, thinly sliced
1 clove minced garlic
2 teaspoons peeled and grated fresh ginger
2 tablespoons soy sauce
1 teaspoon sugar
1/8 teaspoon dark sesame oil
1/2 cup (75 g) chopped or slivered nuts (use almonds, peanuts or cashews)

In a large frying pan or wok, steam the green beans in about 2 cups (500 ml) of water over medium heat for about 6 minutes. Drain the beans and remove them from the pan. Set the beans aside.

In the same pan, heat the oil over medium heat. Add the onion, garlic and ginger. Sauté them for 3 minutes. Mix in the green beans and reduce the heat to low.

In small bowl or jar, mix the soy sauce, sugar, sesame oil and 2 table-spoons of water. Pour the mixture over the beans. Toss well and heat through.

Sprinkle the beans with the nuts before serving.

Sautéed Zucchini

This recipe can be served as a side dish to accompany other foods, or it makes a great topping for pizza. Yet, it is filling enough to serve as a main dish. To make a full meal, serve it with baked potatoes.

3 tablespoons olive oil
2 pounds (1 kg) zucchini, sliced into thin rounds
1/2 cup (75 g) chopped onion
3 tablespoons chopped fresh basil or 1 tablespoon dried basil
1 tablespoon chopped fresh oregano or 1 teaspoon dried oregano
1/4 teaspoon garlic powder
1/4 teaspoon salt
1/4 teaspoon freshly ground black pepper

Heat the oil in a large frying pan or skillet over medium heat. Add the zucchini and onion. Cook them over medium heat for about 5 minutes, or until they are almost tender. Stir in the basil, oregano, garlic powder, salt and pepper. Sauté for another 5 minutes.

Sloppy Joes

Many people think Sloppy Joes should contain hamburger meat. This recipe uses ground turkey or mashed tofu instead of hamburger because, as a rule, Ayurveda does not encourage the use of red meat to balance the doshas (see page 32). Serve with french fries and a small tossed salad.

3 tablespoons ghee or olive oil
³/4 cup (110 g) chopped onion
³/4 cup (75 g) chopped celery
³/4 cup (125 g) chopped green bell pepper
I pound (500 g) ground turkey (vegetarians can substitute I lb/500 g tofu, mashed)
4 medium tomatoes, chopped, or I can (15 oz/475 g) pureed or chopped tomatoes
2 tablespoons prepared yellow mustard
I tablespoon Worcestershire sauce
I tablespoon brown sugar
¹/4 teaspoon garlic powder
¹/2 teaspoon chili powder
¹/2 teaspoon salt
4 whole wheat hamburger buns

Heat the ghee or oil in a large frying pan or skillet over medium heat. Cook the onion, celery and green pepper for about 4 minutes over medium heat. Add the ground turkey (or mashed tofu) and continue to cook for 5 more minutes, stirring frequently with a fork until the meat is browned. Stir in the tomato, mustard, Worcestershire sauce, sugar, garlic powder, chili powder and salt. Blend the mixture well. Cook for about 2 more minutes, or until the mixture is heated through. Serve over hamburger buns.

VARIATION: *Combine the mixture with 4 cups (520 g) of cooked macaroni shells to create what my mother calls "American Chop Suey."*

Chicken with Mustard Marinade

This sweet, sour, tender chicken dish combines well with lots of warm, sweet vegetable side dishes. The mustard and toasted sesame oil add a warming, robust flavor. Serve with baked sweet potatoes and Sautéed Artichoke Hearts (page 58).

$1/4$ cup (50 g) firmly packed brown sugar or $1/4$ cup (65 ml) maple syrup
2 tablespoons Dijon mustard
1 clove garlic, minced, or $1/8$ teaspoon garlic powder
2 tablespoons vinegar
$1/2$ teaspoon dark sesame oil
$1 1/2$ tablespoons soy sauce
4 chicken breasts, skin removed

To prepare the marinade, in a large bowl or baking pan combine the sugar or syrup, mustard, garlic, vinegar, oil and soy sauce. Mix well. Add the chicken to the marinade and coat well. Cover and refrigerate for several hours or overnight.

Heat the oven to 300°F (150°C). Drain off about half of the marinade and set aside. Place the chicken with the remaining marinade in a baking pan. Bake for 45 minutes if the chicken is on the bone, or for 35 minutes if the chicken is boneless. About halfway through the baking time, spoon a tablespoon of marinade over each breast to keep them moist.

Sautéed Artichoke Hearts

1 can (14 oz/400 g) artichoke hearts, drained and rinsed
6 tablespoons butter
¹/₈ teaspoon salt
¹/₈ teaspoon freshly gound black pepper

If the artichoke hearts are frozen, thaw them until they break apart.
Then steam them in 1 cup (250 ml) of water, covered, for 5 minutes.
Melt the butter in a frying pan over medium heat. Add the artichoke
hearts. Sauté them for about 3 minutes. Stir in the salt and pepper.

Chicken Cacciatore

Italian dishes, because they are typically warm and rich, are great for balancing vata. I chose to include this one because it's so easy and delicious. Serve with French bread and Sautéed Zucchini (page 55).

2 tablespoons extra-virgin olive oil
1/2 cup (75 g) chopped onion
1/2 cup (50 g) chopped celery
1 clove garlic, minced
2 cups (500 ml) plain tomato sauce, homemade or bottled
3/4 cup (185 ml) dry sherry or red wine
1 teaspoon dried basil
1/2 teaspoon dried oregano
1 bay leaf
4 chicken breasts, skin removed

Preheat the oven to 300°F (150°C). In a small frying pan, heat the oil over medium heat. Sauté the onion, celery and garlic for about 2 minutes, or until tender. In a bowl, combine the sautéed vegetables (including the pan juices) with the tomato sauce, sherry or wine, basil, oregano and bay leaf. Place the chicken breasts in a baking pan and pour the sauce mixture evenly over the chicken. Bake for 45 minutes if the chicken is on the bone, or for 35 minutes if it is boneless. Remove the bay leaf before serving.

Baked Fish with Herbs

According to Ayurveda, seafood is sweet, heavy and warming—just the thing to counteract too much vata. Perhaps you've heard that fish is good for the nervous system. This recipe combines sweet herbs, salty soy sauce and sour lemon juice with the fish to include all three vata-balancing tastes. Serve with Bulgur Wheat Pilaf (page 66) and Boiled Beets (page 61).

2 tablespoons ghee or butter, melted

2 tablespoons soy sauce

2 teaspoons lemon juice

2 teaspoons dried herbs (choose one or more of the following: parsley, basil, oregano, marjoram, tarragon or dill)

4 mild fish fillets or steaks (about one pound/500 g total) such as flounder, halibut, snapper, salmon, swordfish or grouper

4 very thin slices of onion or 4 tablespoons minced green onion

Preheat the oven to 450°F (230°C). In a small bowl, combine the melted ghee or butter, soy sauce, lemon juice and herbs. Arrange the fish in a baking pan. Drizzle 1 tablespoon of the liquid mixture evenly over each fish fillet or steak. Top each with a slice of onion or 1 tablespoon minced green onion. If there is any liquid left in the bowl, drizzle it over the onion. Bake for 10 minutes per 1-inch (2.5-cm) thickness of fish. For instance, if the fish is 1/2 inch (1.25 cm) thick, bake for 5 minutes; if it is 1 inch (2.5 cm) thick, bake for 10 minutes.

Boiled Beets

I pound (500 g) young beets, unpeeled
2 tablespoons ghee or butter, melted
1/4 teaspoon salt

Place the beets in enough boiling water to cover them. Reduce the heat to a simmer and cook them for 30 minutes. Drain the beets and plunge them into cold water to cool them. After cooling, the skins should easily slip off. Slice the beets or serve them whole if they are very small. Reheat and toss them with the melted ghee or butter and salt before serving.

Salmon Loaf with Rob's Horseradish Sauce

This is one of my favorite dishes for a pot-luck dinner party—people always ask me for this recipe. My husband Rob came up with the tangy sauce, which perfectly complements the sweet and salty salmon loaf. Serve with buttered egg noodles and Candied Carrots (page 63).

I can (14 oz/400 g) salmon (pink or red)
I cup (100 g) breadcrumbs
I tablespoon wheat bran or oat bran
2 tablespoons ghee or butter, melted
I egg, beaten
2 tablespoons chopped fresh parsley or 2 teaspoons dried parsley
¹/₂ teaspoon dried dill
³/₄ cup (185 ml) mayonnaise
I tablespoon Dijon mustard
¹/₂ tablespoon prepared horseradish

Preheat the oven to 350°F (175°C). Drain most of the liquid from the can of salmon. In a large bowl, combine the salmon with the bread-crumbs, bran, ghee or butter, egg, parsley and dill. Flake the fish with a fork to blend all ingredients well. Press this mixture into a lightly greased 1-quart casserole dish or loaf pan. Bake for about 45 min-utes. The loaf should be firm and the top crusty when done.

To make Rob's horseradish sauce: In a small bowl, blend together the mayonnaise, mustard and horseradish. Spoon a desired amount on top of each serving of salmon loaf.

Candied Carrots

4 carrots, sliced in rounds
1/4 teaspoon salt
5 tablespoons ghee or butter
1/4 cup (50 g) firmly packed brown sugar

Cook the carrots in 2 cups (500 ml) of boiling water for about 5 minutes, or until they are tender. Drain the carrots, salt them and set aside. In a frying pan or skillet, melt the ghee or butter over medium heat. Add the sugar and stir until it blends into the butter. Add the carrots and toss them until they are well coated.

Seafood Cakes

Try this recipe using the various seafoods suggested. You'll find each result tasty and satisfying. The cakes can also be served between hamburger buns as seafood burgers. Serve with french fries and a small tossed salad.

2 cups (450 g) flaked cooked fresh seafood (salmon, tuna, codfish, crabmeat or shrimp)
2 eggs, beaten
2 tablespoons mayonnaise
1 cup (175 g) crushed unsalted crackers
1 teaspoon Worcestershire sauce
2 tablespoons chopped fresh parsley or 2 teaspoons dried parsley
1/2 teaspoon dry mustard
3/4 cup (75 g) all-purpose flour
4 tablespoons ghee or butter

In a large bowl, combine the seafood, eggs, mayonnaise, crushed crackers, Worcestershire sauce, parsley and mustard, and mix them well. Form the mixture into 8 patties, about 3 inches (7.5 cm) in diameter. Dust each patty on both sides with flour. To make the patties firmer and easier to fry, cover and refrigerate them for at least an hour. Heat the ghee or butter in a large frying pan or skillet over medium heat until it is melted. Fry the patties for 4 minutes on each side. Serve with lemon wedges, or for a richer taste, serve with tartar sauce.

Scallops in Wine Sauce

Since seafood is a good vata-balancer, why not indulge in some delicate, creamy scallops? This recipe uses an aromatic poaching liquid of wine and herbs. Serve with steamed rice and Steamed Asparagus (page 50).

4 tablespoons ghee or butter
3 tablespoons minced scallion
I teaspoon dried marjoram
I tablespoon chopped fresh parsley or I teaspoon dried parsley
I pound (500 g) large sea scallops
I cup (250 ml) white wine
I tablespoon fresh lemon juice
I teaspoon sugar
I tablespoon cornstarch
Garnish: lemon slices

In a large frying pan or skillet, heat the ghee or butter over medium heat. Add the scallion, marjoram and parsley. Sauté for 2 minutes. Add the scallops and sauté, stirring constantly, for 3 minutes. Add the wine, lemon juice and sugar. Cook for another 3 minutes. Dissolve the cornstarch in 2 tablespoons water, add it to the sauce, and stir until the sauce thickens. Serve garnished with lemon slices.

Bulgur Wheat Pilaf

Bulgur wheat grains have been partially cooked, then dried and cracked into smaller pieces. You should be able to find this flavorful grain in most large supermarkets. This recipe is a suggested side dish to serve with Baked Fish with Herbs (page 60). However, it is hearty enough to serve by itself as a main course. To make a full vegetarian meal, serve it with Baked Winter Squash (page 67).

1½ (375 ml) cups broth (chicken or vegetable)
1 cup (170 g) bulgur wheat, uncooked
2 tablespoons ghee or olive oil
½ cup (75 g) chopped onion
½ cup (50 g) chopped celery
½ cup (50 g) chopped carrot

In a medium saucepan, bring the broth to a boil. Stir the wheat into the boiling broth. Cover the pan, remove from heat, and let it sit for about 30 minutes, until the wheat is tender and the liquid has been absorbed.

Heat the ghee or oil in a large frying pan or skillet. Add the onion, celery and carrot and cook them over medium heat for about 5 minutes, until they are tender. Turn off the heat. Blend the wheat into the cooked vegetables in the frying pan. Turn the heat to medium and cook, stirring well, until the mixture is warmed through.

Baked Winter Squash

1 large or 2 small butternut squash or other winter varieties such as
  acorn squash or turban squash
2 tablespoons ghee or butter
4 tablespoons maple syrup

Preheat the oven to 400°F (200°C). Split the squash in half and
remove the seeds. Place the cut sides down in a baking dish and bake
for about 45 minutes, or until the squash is easily pierced with a
fork. Remove the squash from the oven and evenly spread the ghee
or butter onto the cut sides. Drizzle the squash with the syrup. Bake
for a few more minutes, cut side up.

Oat Bran Muffins

Bananas and raisins sweeten these tasty bran muffins. They can be enjoyed for breakfast or as the grain portion of lunch or supper. To make a full meal, serve them with scrambled eggs and Simple Fruit Salad (page 69).

1/2 cup (50 g) all-purpose flour
1/2 cup (75 g) whole wheat flour
1/2 cup (75 g) oats
I cup (100 g) oat bran
I tablespoon baking powder
1/4 cup (65 ml) molasses
2 bananas, mashed
I cup (250 ml) milk
I egg, beaten
I cup (150 g) raisins

Preheat the oven to 400°F (200°C). In a large bowl, combine the flours, oats, oat bran and baking powder. In another bowl, combine the molasses, bananas, milk and egg. Combine the wet and dry ingredients in the large bowl. Mix them well. Gently stir in the raisins. Spoon the batter into 18 greased muffin cups. Bake for 18 minutes. Let them cool before removing them from the pan.

Simple Fruit Salad

2 large oranges
2 bananas
1/2 cup (40 g) shredded coconut

Peel the oranges and divide them into sections. Slice the bananas into
1/4-inch (6-mm) rounds. Gently mix the oranges and bananas together.
Sprinkle the mixture with the coconut.

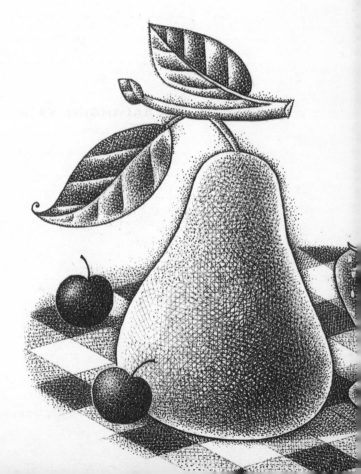

OTHER IDEAS FOR VATA-BALANCING FOODS

Now it's your turn! While reading this chapter on balancing vata with food, I'm sure you thought of some of your favorite vata-balancing recipes. You can list them here under the suggested categories. Use the guidelines on page 40 to make any necessary modifications.

MAIN DISHES FOR BALANCING VATA:

_____

_____

_____

_____

_____

_____

_____

DESSERTS FOR BALANCING VATA:

_____

_____

_____

_____

SNACKS FOR BALANCING VATA:

_____

_____

_____

BEVERAGES FOR BALANCING VATA:

_____

_____

_____

BREAKFAST FOR BALANCING VATA:

_____

_____

_____

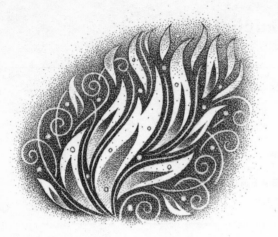

BALANCING PITTA

Pitta is the *fire* principle. It influences the processes of digestion and metabolism. Its basic qualities include being fast moving, hot in temperature, light in weight, wet to the touch, and sour-tasting.

"Double, double,

toil and trouble

Fire burn and

cauldron bubble."

Shakespeare,
MacBeth

SYMPTOMS OF A PITTA IMBALANCE

Heat is the main characteristic of a pitta disorder. A balanced amount is necessary to keep your engine running. But when there is too much pitta in the physiology, your engine will get overheated, and that can spell trouble. You may have a pitta imbalance if you are experiencing one or more of the following symptoms:

- Digestive problems such as heartburn, sour stomach, acid indigestion, ulcers or diarrhea
- Skin inflammation such as rash, acne or hemorrhoids
- Anger, irritability, temper tantrums
- Hot flashes
- Excess sweating
- Bloodshot eyes, not related to allergy

POSSIBLE CAUSES

Pitta is highest in the summer, when the weather is hot. Long periods of exposure to hot weather can bring on a pitta imbalance. Allowing yourself to get sunburned is a surefire way to bring on a pitta imbalance. Or maybe you've been eating too many spicy, fried, sour or salty foods. It could be that your constitution is pitta, making you more vulnerable to pitta-related problems.

WHAT TO EAT

To cool off and balance pitta, eat more foods that taste sweet, bitter and astringent. Emphasizing the sweet taste does not mean gorging on foods loaded with sugar. Foods like milk, bread and ripe fruit are naturally sweet, and are what Ayurveda means by sweet. Eat sugary foods in moderation. A scoop of ice cream will indeed cool you down, but eating a quart of it could bring on a kapha imbalance. Foods to increase and reduce to balance pitta are listed on the following pages. Please don't limit your diet to sweet, bitter and astringent food during this time. Remember to include at least a little of the other tastes to maintain a balance.

Cool Hint: Blasts of heat from a hot oven will not have a very balancing effect on a cook with a pitta imbalance. The recipes in this section do not call for oven baking.

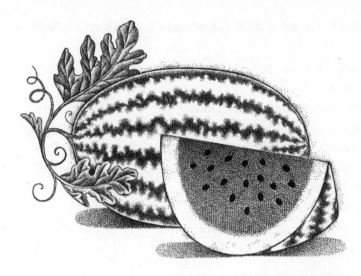

FOODS TO INCREASE (+) WHEN BALANCING PITTA

+ Sweet foods (bread, milk and fruit)
+ Bitter foods (green, leafy vegetables)
+ Astringent foods (lima beans, apples)
+ Cool foods
+ Sweet fruits (grapes, melon, pineapple, berries, prunes, red apples, ripe pears)
+ Vegetables, raw and cooked
+ Legumes (beans, peas and lentils)
+ Wheat and rice
+ Chicken and turkey (especially the white meat)
+ Dairy products (except hard cheeses like cheddar, which tend to be sour)
+ Sweet herbs (mints, fresh coriander (cilantro), dill weed, fennel, fresh basil)

FOODS TO REDUCE (-) WHEN BALANCING PITTA

- Sour foods (fresh lemon juice is an exception; it has a neutral effect on pitta)
- Salty foods (table salt, soy sauce)
- Pungent spices. A little curry powder or dried (not fresh) ginger, however, can actually have a sweet rather than a spicy effect.
- Seafood (except shrimp, which is acceptable in small or moderate amounts)
- Egg yolks
- Tomatoes, hot peppers and raw onion
- Honey
- Nuts
- Oily, greasy, fatty or fried foods
- Red meat

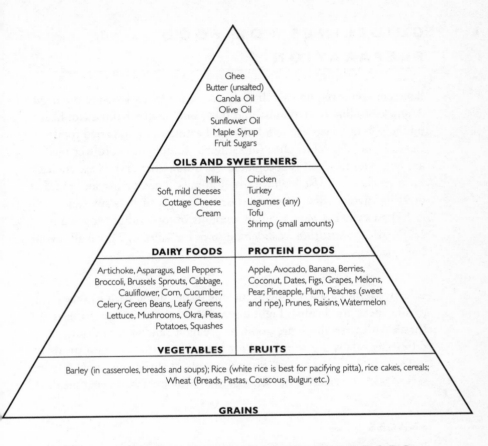

PITTA-PACIFYING PYRAMID OF FOODS

A modified version of the 1992 United States Department of Agriculture's Food Guide Pyramid showing foods that help to balance pitta dosha.

GUIDELINES FOR FOOD PREPARATION

Balancing pitta requires cooling down, so try to avoid using the oven. A quick broiling is okay now and then, but lengthy baking can heat up the whole house. Fats and oils are heating, so avoid fried foods. Use less cooking oil or ghee for sautéing. Canola or sunflower oils are best, and olive oil is acceptable. As usual, ghee is the best choice for a cooking oil. Use lowfat or nonfat milk, mayonnaise and salad dressing. Avoid using salty and sour flavorings, such as soy sauce (salty) and vinegar (sour). Small amounts of low-sodium soy sauce can be used. Substitute fresh lemon juice for vinegar. Above all, avoid hot spices.

Effective pitta-balancing meals include dishes made with legumes (lentils, peas and beans). Light pasta dishes, such as pasta primavera (pasta with vegetables) are good, as are light sandwiches. Cool, refreshing salads are wonderful for balancing pitta. The best meats to use are chicken, turkey and small amounts of shrimp. A cooked grain served with a vegetable or two makes a great pitta-balancing meal.

SNACKS

People with pitta constitutions may sometimes find that a meal has been digested quickly and the stomach is growling for a little "smackerel of something," to quote Winnie-the-Pooh. A juicy piece of fruit, like watermelon or cantaloupe, will quench the flames. Other good pitta-balancing snacks are lowfat cottage cheese, raw veggies, a cookie and cold milk, or low-sodium crackers with a little peanut butter or jelly. I like popcorn with a little melted ghee and washed down with a big glass of fruit juice.

BEVERAGES

A pitta imbalance can often cause excessive thirst, so it's important to drink lots of fluids, especially cold water. Almost all fruit juices are good, especially apple, grape, pineapple, berry and mango. Citrus fruits, such as orange and grapefruit, are too acidic and will elevate pitta. Sweet lemonade, however, has a neutralizing effect. This is a great time to drink fruit smoothies, made by combining lowfat milk with chunks of sweet fruit in a blender. Avoid having icy drinks with a meal. Icy drinks make the stomach contract and this can hinder digestion. Pitta-balancing herbal teas include chamomile, jasmine, lemon balm, peppermint and spearmint.

BREAKFAST

Almost any pitta-balancing breakfast should include sweet fruit. Good breakfasts include French toast, pancakes, cold cereal, toast, muffins or bagels.

It's best to stay away from pastries, since they are usually loaded with fat. Egg yolks will increase pitta, so if you want eggs for breakfast, use egg whites or egg substitute. If you like tofu, try scrambling soft tofu in a little ghee or butter.

DESSERTS

There are lots of desserts that are both sweet and cool. Here's one to really cool you down.

Fruit Sorbet

1/2 cup (100 g) sugar
1/2 cup (125 ml) water or dry, white wine
1 tablespoon fresh lemon juice
3 cups (500 g) coarsely chopped fresh, ripe, sweet fruit (such as banana,
  peach, pear, strawberry, cantaloupe or watermelon)

In a saucepan, mix the sugar, water or wine, and lemon juice. Bring the mixture to a boil. Reduce the heat to low and simmer for about 1 minute until the sugar dissolves. Remove from the heat and set aside to cool.

Puree the fruit in a blender or food processor. Combine the pureed fruit with the sugar mixture, stirring well. Pour this mixture into an 8-inch (20-cm)-square freezer tray. Cover and refrigerate the tray for about 1 hour.

Transfer the tray from the refrigerator to the freezer. After about 30 minutes, the mixture will have started to form a frozen crust. Remove it from the freezer and stir it well with a spoon, breaking up the crust. Place it back in the freezer. Repeat this procedure every 30 minutes during the next 2 hours as it freezes. This mixing process is necessary to ensure a smooth, soft texture—otherwise, you'll end up with a solid block of ice.

It's not too hard to think of cool, sweet desserts. Just remember, all things in moderation! Here are some other pitta-balancing dessert ideas:

- Ice cream, with fruit sauce or chocolate sauce
- Sherbet or sorbet
- Frozen yogurt or frozen tofu-based dessert
- Fruit pie or shortcake, served cool
- Fresh sweet fruit
- Gelatin mold with fruit

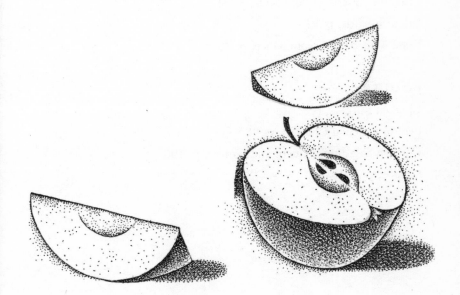

PITTA RECIPES

VEGETABLES

Pea Soup with Spearmint, p. 84

Beans with Rice and Cinnamon, p. 85

Pasta Primavera, p. 87

Sauté of Tofu, p. 88

Stewed Potatoes, p. 90

Herbed Potato Salad, p. 92

Vegetable Burritos, Pitta Style, p. 94

Salad Burritos, p. 95

Pasta with Basil Cream Sauce, p. 96

POULTRY

Chicken Burgers, p. 97

Lemon Poached Chicken, p. 98

Chicken Salad with Curry and Grapes, p. 100

Kebabs, p. 101

SEAFOOD

Poached Shrimp, p. 102

Shrimp Salad in a Pineapple Boat, p. 103

GRAINS

Cool Tabouli Salad, p. 104

Light French Toast, p. 106

SIDE DISHES

Steamed Summer Squash, p. 86

Steamed Green Beans, p. 89

Fruit and Cottage Cheese Salad, p. 91

Succotash, p. 93

Steamed Spinach, p. 99

Steamed Broccoli, p. 105

Pea Soup with Spearmint

Legumes (lentils, peas and beans) have an astringent (drying) quality that works well to balance pitta. This recipe eliminates the ham that is included in traditional pea soup recipes. Spearmint adds an interesting flavor and also a cooling effect. Serve with wheat rolls and a tossed salad.

I cup (225 g) split peas, rinsed and drained
6 cups (1.5 liters) low-sodium broth (chicken or vegetable) or water
I cup (150 g) chopped onion
I cup (150 g) chopped carrot
I cup (100 g) chopped celery
¼ teaspoon salt
¼ teaspoon freshly ground black pepper
3 tablespoons chopped fresh spearmint leaves or I tablespoon dried
   spearmint

Put the peas, water or broth, onion and carrot in a large saucepan or soup pot and bring it to a boil. Reduce the heat to low and simmer, covered, for 1 hour. Add the celery, salt, pepper and spearmint. Simmer for another 15 minutes.

Beans with Rice and Cinnamon

This legume dish is sweet, tasty and very satisfying. It can also be served as a cool salad when chilled and mixed with some chopped avocado and a little canola or sunflower oil. Serve with Steamed Summer Squash (page 86).

1 tablespoon ghee, butter or canola oil
¹/₂ cup (75 g) finely chopped onion
1 cup (225 g) rice, uncooked
2 cups (500 ml) low-sodium broth (chicken or vegetable) or water
1 cinnamon stick
Freshly ground black pepper, to taste
2 cups (500 g) beans, cooked (use red beans, pinto, kidney or black beans)

Heat the ghee, butter or oil in a large frying pan over medium heat. Sauté the onion for about 1 minute, or until tender. Add the rice and stir. Add the water or broth, cinnamon stick and pepper. Bring the mixture to a boil, stir and cover. Reduce the heat to low and simmer for 10 minutes or until the rice is tender and the liquid has been absorbed. Remove the cinnamon stick. Stir in the cooked beans and heat for about 5 more minutes.

Steamed Summer Squash

I pound (500 g) summer squash, cut into ¹/₂-inch (1.25-cm) slices

In a saucepan, bring 1¹/₂ cups (375 ml) of water to a boil. Add the squash, cover the pan and simmer over medium heat for 5 minutes. The squash should be just tender but not mushy. Drain the squash and serve it with a little ghee or butter.

Pasta Primavera

The vegetables suggested in this recipe are all good for balancing pitta. For variety and flavor, I recommend using a little of each of them. To give this dish an Italian flavor, use extra virgin olive oil. Oregano, a traditional Italian herb, is not used because it is too heating. Serve with French bread.

3 tablespoons extra virgin olive oil
1/2 cup (75 g) chopped onion
3 cups (400 to 500 g) assorted fresh vegetables, cut into 1-inch (2.5 cm)
     pieces (such as broccoli, zucchini, summer squash, snow peas, carrots,
     asparagus, sweet red bell pepper and mushrooms)
1 tablespoon chopped fresh basil or 1 teaspoon dried basil
1 tablespoon chopped fresh parsley or 1 teaspoon dried parsley
1/4 teaspoon salt
Freshly ground black pepper, to taste
1 pound (500 g) pasta, cooked (preferably angel hair or linguini)
4 tablespoons grated Parmesan cheese

Heat the oil in a large frying pan or wok over medium heat. Cook the onion for about one minute, or until tender. Add the vegetables and sauté for about 5 minutes. Stir in the basil, parsley, salt and pepper. Gently stir in the cooked pasta and toss it with the vegetables until it is well-mixed and heated through. Sprinkle each serving with one tablespoon of grated Parmesan cheese.

Sauté of Tofu

For some reason, many nonvegetarians can't say the word tofu with a straight face. Tofu is soy bean curd, and it's a great protein food. It is found in two varieties, firm and soft. It has a neutral flavor when eaten plain, so it needs to be cooked with flavorful ingredients. In this recipe, I use a flavorful marinade. This is easy to prepare, and it tastes great. Serve it with steamed rice and Steamed Green Beans (opposite).

1 package (16 oz/500 g) firm tofu
1 cup (250 ml) apple or pineapple juice
2 tablespoons low-sodium soy sauce
1/4 teaspoon powdered ginger
2 tablespoons ghee, butter or canola oil

Drain the tofu and slice it lengthwise into 4 thin slices. In a glass baking dish, mix the juice, soy sauce and ginger. Place the tofu slices side by side in the marinade mixture and refrigerate for a few hours or overnight. Remove the tofu from the marinade and carefully pat it dry with a paper towel. Heat the ghee, butter or oil in a large frying pan. Sauté the tofu over medium heat for 2 or 3 minutes on each side.

VARIATION: *This marinated tofu is also good cut into 1-inch (2.5-cm) cubes and stir-fried with vegetables.*

Steamed Green Beans

1 pound (500 g) green beans, trimmed (use Blue Lakes, pole beans, sugar snaps or snow pea pods)

Bring 1¹/2 cups (375 ml) of water to a boil. Add the beans and cover the pan. Cook over medium heat for about 10 minutes, or until the beans are just tender. Drain and serve.

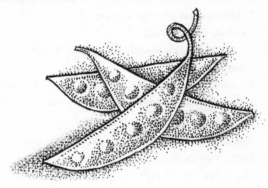

Stewed Potatoes

This recipe makes a nice side dish, but is filling enough to serve as a main dish. White potatoes are great for balancing pitta, as long as they are not fried. Serve with Fruit and Cottage Cheese Salad (page 91) and rye bread.

6 medium red potatoes or 12 small red potatoes
2 tablespoons ghee or butter
I onion, thinly sliced
I cup (250 ml) low-sodium chicken broth
I bay leaf
2 tablespoons chopped fresh parsley or 2 teaspoons dried parsley
I teaspoon snipped fresh dill or 1/2 teaspoon dried dill

Rinse and scrub the potatoes, leaving the skins on. Cut the potatoes into 1/4-inch (6-mm) slices. Heat the ghee or butter over medium heat in a large frying pan. Add the onion slices and sauté for about 1 minute, or until they are tender. Add the potato slices, broth and bay leaf. Cover and cook over medium-low heat for 10 minutes. Remove the cover. Sprinkle the parsley and dill evenly over the potatoes. Turn the heat up to medium and cook, uncovered, for 5 minutes. Remove the bay leaf before serving.

Fruit and Cottage Cheese Salad

2 large pears or peaches
4 large lettuce leaves
2 cups (450 g) lowfat cottage cheese
2 tablespoons lowfat mayonnaise
4 cherries, strawberries or raspberries

Peel the skin from the fruit. Cut both pieces of fruit in half. Scoop out the seeds to form a hollow in each half. Place the fruit half on a lettuce leaf, on a small plate. Place 1/2 cup (110 g) of the cottage cheese onto the center of each fruit half, and 1/2 tablespoon of mayonnaise on top of the cottage cheese. Set a cherry or berry on top of the mayonnaise.

Herbed Potato Salad

Fresh herbs flavor this cooling salad. Summer is the best time to make this version of potato salad because that's when fresh herbs are so plentiful. Serve with Succotash (page 93).

2 pounds (1 kg) red potatoes, unpeeled
1/2 cup (50 g) chopped celery
2 tablespoons chopped fresh parsley
1 tablespoon chopped fresh spearmint leaves
1 tablespoon chopped fresh basil
1 tablespoon snipped fresh dill
1/2 cup (125 g) plain yogurt, lowfat or nonfat
1/2 cup (110 g) lowfat mayonnaise
1 tablespoon fresh lemon juice
1 tablespoon honey or sugar

Rinse and scrub the potatoes. Place them in enough boiling water to cover all of the potatoes. Cover the pan and cook them over medium heat for 15 to 25 minutes, depending upon their size. A fork should easily pass into the potatoes when they are cooked, but they should not be mushy. Drain the potatoes and rinse them with cold water to stop the cooking action. When the potatoes are cool, chop them into 1/2-inch (1.25-cm) pieces.

In a large bowl, combine the chopped potatoes with the celery, parsley, spearmint, basil and dill. Set this mixture aside.

In a small bowl, combine the yogurt, mayonnaise, lemon juice and honey or sugar. Pour this sauce over the potatoes and gently mix. Chill before serving.

Succotash

1 1/2 cups (250 g) fresh or frozen corn kernels, cooked
1 1/2 cups (275 g) fresh or frozen lima beans, cooked
2 tablespoons ghee or butter
1/2 cup (125 ml) lowfat milk or cream
Salt and freshly ground black pepper, to taste

Combine the corn, lima beans, ghee or butter, and milk or cream in a saucepan. Cook, stirring occasionally, over medium heat for 3 to 5 minutes, or until it is heated through. Season the mixture with a little salt and pepper.

Vegetable Burritos, Pitta Style

This version of burritos is sweet and cool. Mild white cheese is used instead of cheddar, which is too sour. Crushed pineapple replaces the spicy salsa. Cooling fresh coriander adds an interesting herb flavor. Served with a tossed salad.

4 tablespoons ghee, butter or canola oil
I pound (500 g) summer squash or zucchini, chopped
I pound (500 g) broccoli, chopped
I cup (70 g) chopped mushrooms
4 tablespoons chopped fresh coriander leaves (cilantro)
4 flour tortillas (about 8 in/20 cm in diameter)
2 cups (225 g) shredded mild white cheese (such as mozzarella, farmer, or Havarti)
1/2 cup (125 ml) crushed pineapple

Heat the ghee or oil over medium heat in a large frying pan or skillet. Add the squash and broccoli. Sauté the vegetables over medium heat for about 5 minutes. Add the mushrooms and fresh coriander. Sauté this for an additional minute and turn the heat to low.

To prepare the tortillas, melt 1/4 teaspoon ghee or butter in a small frying pan over medium heat. Place one tortilla in the pan and sprinkle 1/2 cup (55 g) of cheese evenly over the tortilla. Heat the tortilla over medium-low heat until the cheese melts. Remove the tortilla to a plate and spoon one quarter of the vegetable mixture onto half of the tortilla. Spread 2 tablespoons of the crushed pineapple over the vegetables and fold the empty half of the tortilla over the full half.

Salad Burritos

Here's another cool burrito, crunchy on the inside, soft on the outside. Serve them with Corn on the Cob (page 47).

BURRITOS:

4 flour tortillas (about 8 in/20 cm in diameter)
4 sandwich-size slices of mild white cheese (such as mozzarella, farmer
    or Havarti) or thin slices of smoked turkey luncheon meat
1/2 pound (250 g) squash or zucchini, chopped
I cup (70 g) chopped mushrooms
1/2 cup (55 g) shredded carrot
4 tablespoons chopped fresh coriander leaves (cilantro)
I cup (55 g) shredded lettuce
I cup (35 g) alfalfa sprouts

GUACAMOLE:

2 medium avocados, mashed
2 tablespoons lowfat mayonnaise or plain yogurt
I teaspoon fresh lemon juice
I tablespoon chopped fresh coriander leaves (cilantro)

To prepare the guacamole: Mix together the mashed avocado, mayonnaise or yogurt, lemon juice and the 1 tablespoon fresh coriander.

To prepare the burritos: Slightly heat them between sheets of wax paper in a microwave oven, or steam them on a rack in a pan with a little water. They should be soft and pliable, but not gooey. Place one tortilla each on four plates. Spread each tortilla with 1/4 cup (60 g) guacamole. Place one slice of cheese on top of the guacamole. Set the plates aside.

In a bowl, combine the squash, mushrooms, carrot and fresh coriander. Spoon one quarter of this mixture onto half of each tortilla. Then top each tortilla with 1/4 cup (12 g) shredded lettuce and 1/4 cup (8 g) sprouts. Fold the empty halves of the tortillas over the full halves and they are ready to eat.

Pasta with Basil Cream Sauce

Fresh basil, used in moderation, is good for balancing pitta. Actually, it is effective in balancing all three doshas. This delicious, creamy sauce can also be served over baked potatoes or cooked vegetables such as broccoli, Brussels sprouts or cauliflower. Serve with tossed salad.

3 tablespoons ghee or butter
3 tablespoons all-purpose flour
1 1/2 cups (375 ml) lowfat milk
2 tablespoons chopped scallions
1/2 cup (20 g) chopped fresh basil
1 pound (500 g) pasta, cooked (preferably angel hair or linguini)

Melt the ghee or butter in a saucepan over medium heat. Quickly blend in the flour, stirring well with a fork to prevent lumping. Gradually pour in the milk, stirring with a whisk to keep the mixture smooth. When the sauce has thickened, remove it from the heat.

Coat a small frying pan with canola oil or cooking oil spray and heat to medium. Sauté the scallions for about 1 minute, until they are tender. Add the scallions and basil leaves to the cream sauce. Reheat the sauce over medium heat for a minute or so, mixing well, until it is heated through. Spoon the sauce over the cooked pasta.

Chicken Burgers

These lowfat burgers are great for a summer cookout, or they can be broiled in the oven. Serve them with sliced avocado, lettuce, alfalfa sprouts and lowfat mayonnaise, if desired. They go great with Herbal Potato Salad (page 92).

1 pound (500 g) ground chicken or turkey
1 cup (100 g) breadcrumbs, dry and unseasoned
2 tablespoons chopped scallions
2 tablespoons maple syrup
1 tablespoon lemon juice
2 teaspoons Worcestershire sauce
1/8 teaspoon salt
4 hamburger buns

In a large bowl, thoroughly mix the chicken, breadcrumbs, scallions, syrup, lemon juice, Worcestershire sauce and salt. Shape the mixture into four round patties. Grill the patties over hot coals for about 5 minutes on each side, making sure they are no longer pink inside. Or, broil them on a broiler pan in the oven for about 5 minutes on each side. Again, they should not be pink inside. Serve them on the hamburger buns.

Lemon Poached Chicken

Citrus juices, being acidic, tend to increase pitta. However, fresh lemon juice is an exception. It has a neutral effect. Combined with sugar and fresh coriander, it makes a light, refreshing poaching liquid. Serve with steamed rice and Steamed Spinach (page 99).

I tablespoon ghee or butter
2 tablespoons fresh lemon juice
I tablespoon sugar
4 tablespoons chopped onion or scallion
I red bell pepper, cut into thin strips
I tablespoon chopped fresh coriander leaves (cilantro) or I teaspoon ground coriander
4 boneless, skinless chicken breasts
I cup (70 g) sliced mushrooms
I tablespoon cornstarch

Place the ghee or butter, lemon juice, sugar and 1/2 cup (125 ml) water in a large skillet or Dutch oven. Heat this until just boiling. Add the onion, pepper strips, coriander and chicken breasts. Cover the pan and simmer over medium-low heat for 8 minutes. Add the mushrooms. Cover and simmer for another 3 minutes. Turn the heat to medium. Dissolve the cornstarch in 2 tablespoons of water and cook uncovered, stirring until the sauce thickens.

Steamed Spinach

2 pounds (1 kg) spinach

Rinse the spinach leaves well and remove the tough stems. In a large pot, bring 2 cups (500 ml) of water to a boil. Add the spinach, cover the pot and cook over medium-high heat for about 3 minutes. Drain the spinach well and toss it with a little ghee or butter if desired.

Chicken Salad with Curry and Grapes

This refreshing, tasty salad will really cool you down! Curry powder in small amounts is not heating. Serve with raw veggies such as carrot and celery sticks, and unsalted crackers.

1 cup (220 g) lowfat mayonnaise
1 teaspoon curry powder
4 cups (500 g) chopped cooked chicken
1 cup (175 g) red or green seedless grapes, cut in half
Lettuce leaves

Blend the mayonnaise with the curry powder. Mix this with the chicken and grapes. Serve the chicken mixture on a bed of lettuce.

VARIATION: *Use only 2 cups (250 g) of chicken and add 2 cups (400 g) of cooked pasta shells.*

Kebabs

This recipe is fun to make and to eat. The instructions call for broiling, but the kebabs can also be cooked on an outdoor grill. Serve with steamed rice or couscous.

$^1/_2$ cup (125 ml) pineapple juice
2 tablespoons canola oil
$^1/_4$ teaspoon dark sesame oil
1 tablespoon low-sodium soy sauce
1 tablespoon chopped fresh basil or 1 teaspoon dried basil
2 tablespoons chopped fresh spearmint or peppermint leaves or
    2 teaspoons dried mint
1 teaspoon curry powder
$^1/_4$ teaspoon freshly ground black pepper
2 pounds (1 kg) assorted raw items, cut into 1-inch (2.5-cm) pieces
    (such as chicken, turkey, peeled shrimp, peeled eggplant, partially
    cooked sweet potato, bell pepper, sweet onion, zucchini, summer
    squash, mushroom caps and fresh pineapple)

To make a basting sauce: Mix the juice, oils, soy sauce and spices in a bowl.

Arrange the meat and vegetable pieces alternately on skewers. Baste each skewer with the sauce. Place them on a broiler rack. Place the rack 5 inches from the heat in a preheated broiler. Broil them for about 6 minutes on each side, basting and turning the skewers once. Instead of broiling, they may also be grilled over hot coals for 5 minutes on each side.

Poached Shrimp

Most seafood is warming and rich, and therefore is not good for balancing pitta. Shrimp, however, when eaten in small or moderate amounts, has a neutral effect on pitta. This recipe results in mildly seasoned shrimp that is delicious served warm or chilled. Serve with Stewed Potatoes (page 90) and Steamed Asparagus (page 50).

¹/₄ cup (65 ml) lemon juice
I bay leaf
2 tablespoons chopped scallion
I cup (100 g) chopped celery
10 peppercorns, crushed
I pound (500 g) medium shrimp, shelled

In a large pot, boil 2 cups (500 ml) of water. Add the lemon juice, bay leaf, scallion, celery and peppercorns. Simmer this mixture for 2 minutes. Add the shrimp and simmer for about 2 minutes, or until the shrimp has turned uniformly pink. Serve them immediately, or chill and serve.

Shrimp Salad in a Pineapple Boat

Poached Shrimp (opposite) can be used to make this refreshing salad.
It's very attractive served in a cored pineapple half. Serve with toasted
pita bread or unsalted crackers.

1 cup (220 g) lowfat mayonnaise
1 tablespoon lemon juice
1 teaspoon snipped fresh dill or $^1/_2$ teaspoon dried dill
2 tablespoons chopped fresh parsley or 2 teaspoons dried parsley
4 cups (900 g) chopped cooked shrimp
2 fresh pineapples, halved and cored

In a large bowl, mix the mayonnaise, lemon juice, dill and parsley.
Add the cooked shrimp and mix well. Spoon 1 cup (275 g) of the
mixture into each pineapple half.

Cool Tabouli Salad

Tabouli is a traditional Middle Eastern salad made with cooked grain, usually bulgur wheat. Couscous may be used instead of bulgur wheat. This tabouli recipe omits the traditional raw onion and tomatoes, both of which increase pitta. Instead, it includes cucumber and raisins to increase the cooling effect of the grain and herbs. Serve with lowfat cottage cheese and Steamed Broccoli (opposite).

2 cups (500 g) bulgur wheat, cooked
I cup (25 g) chopped fresh parsley
1/2 cup (15 g) chopped spearmint leaves or I tablespoon dried
    spearmint
1/2 cup (75 g) peeled and chopped cucumber
1/4 cup (35 g) raisins
1/4 cup (65 ml) canola oil
2 tablespoons fresh lemon juice
I teaspoon sugar
4 large lettuce leaves

In a large bowl, combine the bulgur wheat, parsley, spearmint, cucumber and raisins. Mix the ingredients well. Combine the oil, lemon juice and sugar in a jar. Cover and shake well to mix the dressing. Pour the dressing evenly over the salad and toss. Serve the tabouli on the lettuce leaves.

Steamed Broccoli

1 pound (500 g) broccoli, rinsed

Remove and discard the tough parts of the broccoli stems. Cut the broccoli into about 8 spears (florets with stems about 2 in/5 cm long). In a large saucepan, bring 1¹/₂ cups (375 ml) of water to a boil. Add the broccoli and cover the pan. Cook over medium heat for about 5 minutes, until the broccoli is just tender. Drain, and serve with a little ghee or butter if desired.

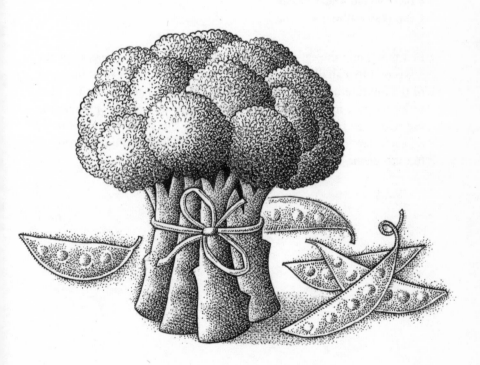

Light French Toast

This simple meal is great for breakfast, lunch or supper. Since egg yolks elevate pitta, this recipe uses only the whites. Serve with fresh fruit and slices of mild white cheese, such as farmer or Havarti.

4 egg whites
4 tablespoons lowfat milk
$1/8$ teaspoon cinnamon
$1/8$ teaspoon nutmeg
I tablespoon ghee or butter
4 slices whole wheat bread
I cup (250 ml) maple syrup

In a bowl, mix the egg whites, milk, cinnamon and nutmeg. Pour the mixture into a shallow pie pan. Let each slice of bread soak up some of the mixture until all sides the bread are well coated. Heat the ghee or butter over medium heat in an extra-large frying pan or skillet (or use two large frying pans). Cook the bread slices for about 2 minutes on each side, or until they are lightly toasted brown. Pour $1/4$ cup (65 ml) of the syrup over each slice of French toast.

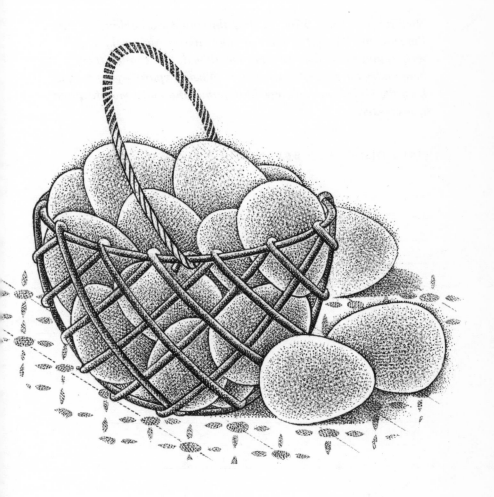

OTHER IDEAS FOR PITTA-BALANCING FOODS

*Now it's your turn! While reading this chapter on balancing pitta,
I'm sure you thought of some of your favorite pitta-balancing
recipes and foods that were not mentioned. You can list them
here under the suggested categories. When preparing your recipes,
keep the Guidelines on page 78 in mind, and make modifications
if necessary.*

MAIN DISHES FOR BALANCING PITTA:

_____

_____

_____

_____

_____

_____

_____

DESSERTS FOR BALANCING PITTA:

_____

_____

_____

SNACKS FOR BALANCING PITTA:

_____

_____

_____

BEVERAGES FOR BALANCING PITTA:

_____

_____

_____

BREAKFASTS FOR BALANCING PITTA:

_____

_____

_____

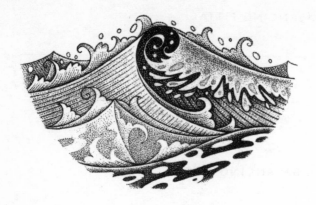

BALANCING KAPHA

Kapha is the water dosha. It provides lubrication and also structure to the cells and tissues of the body. Its basic qualities include being slow-moving, cold in temperature, heavy in weight, wet to the touch and sweet-tasting.

"Day after day,
*   day after day*
We stuck, nor
*   breath nor*
*   motion*
As idle as a
*   painted ship*
Upon a painted ocean."

Samuel Taylor Coleridge,
The Rime of the Ancient Mariner

SYMPTOMS OF A KAPHA IMBALANCE

Having too much kapha in your body is the opposite of having too much vata. Whereas a vata imbalance is characterized by too much movement happening in the physiology, a kapha imbalance will make you feel as if there is too little movement. You feel lethargic, dull and heavy.

If you are experiencing one or more of the following symptoms, you may have a kapha imbalance:

• Sinus congestion, sinus headache, hay fever or stuffy nose
• Headcold or bronchitis
• Lethargy, drowsiness or heavy and prolonged sleep
• Slow digestion, a feeling of fullness and incomplete digestion
• An oppressive feeling, perhaps some mild depression
• Excessively oily skin and scalp
• Weight gain and/or water retention

POSSIBLE CAUSES

Perhaps the weather has been cold and damp and you're feeling that way also—cold, heavy and damp. Typical kapha season for most of the United States is late winter and early spring. Maybe you've been eating too many rich foods or sweets. Or maybe your constitution is such that you naturally have a high proportion of kapha in your physiology, making you prone to occasional kapha-related disorders.

WHAT TO EAT

Whatever the cause, now is the time to eat mostly kapha-balancing foods—those that have the predominant tastes of pungent (spicy), bitter or astringent (drying). The following pages list foods to increase and reduce in your diet to balance kapha. But please do not eat only kapha-balancing foods to the exclusion of all others. Remember, Ayurveda says to include all six tastes in the diet (sweet, sour, salty, bitter, pungent and astringent) to maintain balance.

FOODS TO INCREASE (+) WHEN BALANCING KAPHA

+ Pungent (spicy) foods, such as dishes made with hot peppers
+ Bitter foods, such as leafy green vegetables
+ Astringent (drying) foods, such as apples and peas
+ Warm foods
+ Legumes (beans, peas and lentils)
+ Apples, pears and dried fruits, such as raisins and dried figs
+ Green, leafy vegetables (spinach, collards, broccoli)
+ Fresh corn
+ Chicken and turkey
+ Honey, not cooked
+ Herbs and spices (all of them)

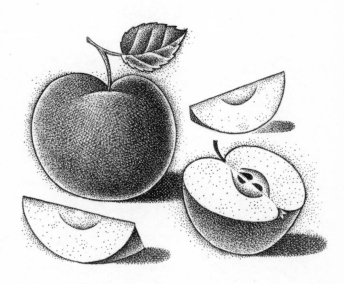

FOODS TO REDUCE (-) WHEN BALANCING KAPHA

- Sweet foods (bananas) and sweeteners (except honey)
- Salty foods, such as table salt or soy sauce
- Sour foods, such as citrus fruits
- Cold foods
- Oily, greasy or fried foods, such as fried chicken
- Seafood (spicy shrimp dishes are okay)
- Red meat
- Dairy products
- Wheat
- Nuts

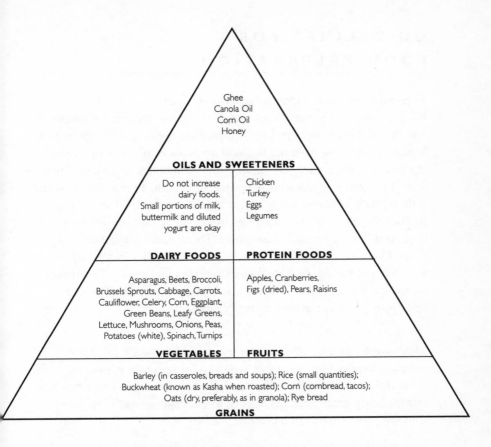

Ghee
Canola Oil
Corn Oil
Honey

OILS AND SWEETENERS

Do not increase dairy foods. Small portions of milk, buttermilk and diluted yogurt are okay	Chicken Turkey Eggs Legumes
DAIRY FOODS	**PROTEIN FOODS**
Asparagus, Beets, Broccoli, Brussels Sprouts, Cabbage, Carrots, Cauliflower, Celery, Corn, Eggplant, Green Beans, Leafy Greens, Lettuce, Mushrooms, Onions, Peas, Potatoes (white), Spinach, Turnips	Apples, Cranberries, Figs (dried), Pears, Raisins
VEGETABLES	**FRUITS**

Barley (in casseroles, breads and soups); Rice (small quantities);
Buckwheat (known as Kasha when roasted); Corn (cornbread, tacos);
Oats (dry, preferably, as in granola); Rye bread

GRAINS

KAPHA-PACIFYING PYRAMID OF FOODS

A modified version of the 1992 United States Department of Agriculture's Food Guide Pyramid showing foods that help to balance kapha dosha.

GUIDELINES FOR
FOOD PREPARATION

Kapha qualities are coldness, heaviness and wetness. Therefore, to balance kapha, use ingredients and cooking methods that promote warmth, lightness and dryness. Appropriate cooking methods include baking, broiling or sautéing in small amounts of oil. The best cooking oils to use are ghee, canola or corn oil. As often as possible, use lowfat or nonfat ingredients. Use little or no salt. Low-sodium substitutions, such as herbs and spices, can make up for the lack of salt. Reduce the use of wheat in recipes by replacing half of the wheat flour with barley or buckwheat flour. These flours are lighter and dryer. Use soba (buckwheat) noodles or rice noodles instead of wheat-based pastas. Be liberal in using herbs and spices. They make up for the loss of flavor in lowfat, low-sodium recipes. If you like spicy food, now is the time to really indulge!

Meals containing legumes (lentils, peas and beans) are great for reducing kapha. Poultry dishes are good for reducing kapha, but only if the skin is removed and they are served without gravy or other rich sauces. Leafy green vegetables, such as cabbage, spinach and broccoli, are good kapha balancers.

The main thing to remember when reducing kapha is to eat on the light side. This means eating foods that are not heavy or rich and always eat in moderation.

SNACKS

Because you're trying to keep your diet light while balancing kapha, snacking is not recommended. But, if there is a need to snack, think in terms of lowfat snacks like dry popcorn, celery and carrot sticks, and lowfat crackers. Apples, pears and dried fruits are good. Unsalted tortilla chips with salsa or spicy bean dip make a good kapha-reducing snack.

BEVERAGES

The best fruit juices for reducing kapha are apple and cranberry. To cut down on the sweetness, dilute fruit juices with water. Hot black coffee is a good kapha-reducing drink. All hot teas are good, especially ginger. See the ginger tea recipe, page 41.

BREAKFAST

Kapha is at its highest during the morning hours, between 6 A.M. and 10 A.M. Since one of the qualities of kapha is heaviness, eating a heavy breakfast could have an unpleasant effect. So, when it comes to breakfast, think extra light when trying to balance kapha. Coffee or tea (caffeinated) will help get you jump-started in the morning. Some good breakfast ideas are oatbread toast or a corn muffin with apple butter or honey, rice crackers with lowfat peanut butter and some raisins, toasted granola with a little lowfat milk, stewed figs, prunes or apples, or some hominy grits drizzled with honey instead of butter.

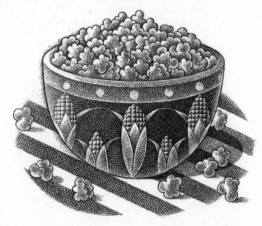

DESSERTS

Sweet flavors increase kapha, so if you're having a problem with kapha, it's best to avoid sweets and desserts. But let's face it, very few people can cut out sweets altogether. Here is a sweet dessert to enjoy that won't worsen a kapha imbalance if eaten in moderation.

Baked, Stuffed Apples

4 tart apples
¹/₄ cup (50 g) firmly packed brown sugar or ¹/₄ cup (65 ml) maple syrup
1 teaspoon ground cinnamon
Pinch of powdered ginger
Pinch of ground cloves
2 tablespoons raisins
¹/₂ cup (125 ml) ginger ale

Preheat the oven to 350°F (175°C). Wash the apples; remove the cores, leaving the bottoms of the apples intact. In a small bowl, combine the sugar or syrup, cinnamon, ginger, cloves and raisins. Fill each apple center with this mixture. Place the stuffed apples in a lightly greased baking pan. Pour the ginger ale into the pan. Bake them for about 40 minutes, basting the apples a few times with the pan juices.

Here are some other desserts that are acceptable when balancing kapha:

- Apple pie or apple "crisp"
- Oatmeal raisin cookies
- Ginger snaps
- Dark chocolate (semisweet is best)

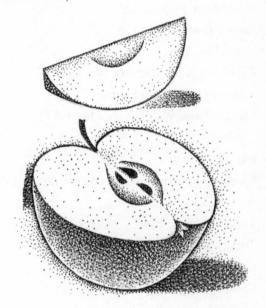

KAPHA RECIPES

GRAINS

SIDE DISHES

Bean Tacos

Refried beans, or *frijoles refritos,* is a Mexican staple food that can be eaten plain or used in a variety of dishes. Here's a basic recipe for refried beans and one of the many ways to use it. Serve with Corn on the Cob (page 47).

Please note: While most people use cheese and/or sour cream on tacos, these two dairy products should not be used in kapha-balancing recipes.

1 tablespoon ghee or canola oil
1/2 cup (75 g) chopped onion
1 clove garlic, minced
2 cups (500 g) beans, cooked (red beans, chili beans or pinto beans)
4 large corn taco shells
2 cups (150 g) shredded lettuce
1 cup (200 g) chopped tomatoes
4 tablespoons taco sauce or salsa (as spicy as desired)

To prepare the beans: Heat the ghee or oil in a large frying pan over medium heat. Add the onion and garlic. Sauté them for about 1 minute, or until they are tender. Turn off the heat. Mash the beans well in a bowl with an electric mixer, large fork or spoon or a potato masher. Add the mashed beans to the cooked onion and garlic in the frying pan. Cook over medium heat, stirring well, until the beans are heated through.

To prepare the shells: Bake them in the oven at 350°F (175 °C), until they are crisp, about 3 minutes. Gently spoon 1/2 cup (140 g) of the refried beans into each shell. Then gently add one quarter of the lettuce and tomatoes into each shell. Place at least 1 tablespoon of taco sauce or salsa on top of the tomatoes.

Spicy Beans 'n' Rice

This quick and easy "red beans 'n' rice" recipe is a light version of a Southern favorite. Serve with Sautéed Greens with Herbs (page 128).

1 tablespoon ghee or canola oil
¹/₂ cup (75 g) chopped onion
1 clove garlic, minced
1 cup (225 g) uncooked rice
2 cups (500 ml) low-sodium broth (chicken or vegetable) or water
2 cups (500 g) beans, cooked (red beans, pinto beans or kidney beans)
¹/₂ teaspoon red pepper flakes or 1/4 teaspoon cayenne powder
1 teaspoon curry powder

Heat the ghee or oil over medium heat in a large frying pan. Add the onion and garlic, and sauté for about 1 minute, or until they are tender. Add the uncooked rice and stir. Add the water or broth. Bring this to a boil, then stir and cover the pan. Simmer the rice over medium heat for 10 minutes, or until it is tender and the liquid has been absorbed. Stir in the beans, red pepper or cayenne, and curry powder. Heat the mixture for a few more minutes and serve.

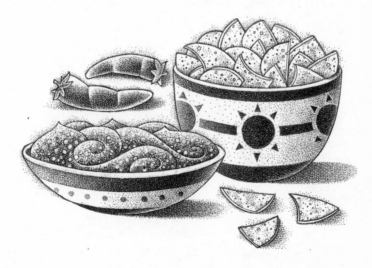

Black Bean Soup

If you like black beans extra spicy, add a second teaspoon of chopped hot peppers to this easy, delicious recipe. Serve with unsalted crackers and carrot sticks.

1 tablespoon ghee or canola oil
1/2 cup (75 g) chopped onion
1/4 cup (25 g) chopped celery
1 teaspoon chopped hot peppers, such as chiles or jalapeños
2 cups (350 g) black beans, cooked
1 cup (200 g) chopped tomatoes
4 cups (1 liter) low-sodium broth (chicken or vegetable)
1 tablespoon wine vinegar (rice wine vinegar works well, but any wine
   vinegar will do)

Heat the ghee or oil in a medium-sized saucepan over medium heat. Add the onion, celery and peppers. Sauté them for about 3 minutes, or until they are tender. Add the black beans, tomatoes and broth. Reduce the heat and simmer for 10 minutes. Stir in the vinegar and serve.

Savory Lentils

This recipe is delicious and versatile. Serve these lentils over soba (buckwheat) noodles, rice or a baked potato, or use them to fill tacos. To round out the meal, serve a tossed salad with lowfat dressing.

1 tablespoon canola oil
1/2 cup (75 g) chopped onion
1/2 cup (50 g) chopped carrot
2 tablespoons chopped fresh herbs or 2 teaspoons dried herbs
   (rosemary, marjoram, savory or thyme)
2 cups (500 ml) lowfat broth (chicken or vegetable)
1 cup (225 g) uncooked lentils
1 can (15 oz/475 ml) tomato sauce
1 cup (250 ml) red wine

In a soup pot or Dutch oven, heat the oil over medium heat. Sauté the onion and carrot for about 3 minutes. Add the herbs and sauté for 1 minute. Add the broth, lentils, tomato sauce and wine. Simmer for 1 hour.

Vegetable Curry

The first step in this recipe is to make a basic curry sauce. The vegetables are then cooked in the sauce, making them very succulent and spicy. You can, however, serve the sauce on precooked vegetables, chicken or shrimp. Serve with steamed rice.

1 tablespoon ghee or canola oil
1 teaspoon whole mustard seeds
1 1/2 tablespoons curry powder
1 clove garlic, minced
One 1/2-inch (1.25-cm) slice
  fresh ginger, peeled and
  minced
1 teaspoon turmeric
2 cups chopped tomatoes,
  or 1 can (15 oz/475 g)
  tomatoes, not drained
1 teaspoon sugar
6 cups (800 to 950 g) assorted raw
  vegetables, chopped into 1-inch pieces
  (Choose from potatoes, carrots, eggplant, green beans, broccoli,
  cauliflower, zucchini and summer squash.)

To make the curry sauce: In a large frying pan or kettle, heat the ghee or oil over medium heat. Add the mustard seeds, curry powder, garlic, ginger and turmeric. Sauté until the seeds start to pop, about 1 minute. Add the tomatoes and sugar. Heat this mixture, stirring, for about 1 minute.

Stir the vegetables into the curry sauce. Cover the pan and cook them over medium heat for 10 minutes. Stir well and reduce the heat to low. Simmer, uncovered, for 15 minutes, stirring occasionally. The vegetables should be tender, but not overcooked, and the sauce should be somewhat thick.

Baked Eggplant Mediterranean

If you've ever sautéed eggplant, you know how much it soaks up the oil. Eggplant is good for balancing kapha, but oily eggplant is not. In this recipe, the eggplant is first boiled until partially cooked, and then baked in a tasty sauce. Serve with soba (buckwheat) noodles.

I large eggplant
I tablespoon ghee or canola oil
1/4 cup (35 g) chopped onion
I clove garlic, minced
I sweet red bell pepper, cut into strips
4 tablespoons tomato paste
1/2 cup (125 ml) water
2 tablespoons pine nuts
I teaspoon turmeric
1/2 teaspoon sugar
1/2 teaspoon ground cinnamon

To prepare the eggplant: Fill a large saucepan two-thirds full of water and bring it to a boil. Cut off the stem end of the eggplant and discard. Place the eggplant in the boiling water. Turn the heat to medium and simmer the eggplant for 15 minutes.

Heat the oil in a large frying pan or skillet over medium heat. Add the onion, garlic and pepper strips. Sauté them for 3 minutes. Turn off the heat and set the pan aside.

Place the tomato paste, water, pine nuts, turmeric, sugar and cinnamon in a blender. Puree for 1 minute or until the mixture is smooth. Add this sauce to the vegetables in the pan and mix well.

Preheat the oven to 350°F (175°C). After the eggplant has cooked for 15 minutes, remove it from the water. Slice it into 1/4-inch (6-mm) rounds. Place a single layer of eggplant rounds in an 8 x 12-inch (20 x 30-cm) baking pan. Spoon the vegetables and sauce evenly over the eggplant slices. Bake for 30 minutes.

Sautéed Greens with Herbs

This recipe makes a great side dish when served with almost any meal that features legumes (beans) or chicken. It works best with fresh spinach, beet greens, turnip greens or Swiss chard. Serve with baked potatoes and rye bread.

2 tablespoons ghee or canola oil
I small onion, thinly sliced
1/4 teaspoon dried oregano
1/4 teaspoon dried basil
2 pounds (I kg) greens (washed, trimmed and chopped)
2 tablespoons wine vinegar

Heat the ghee or oil in a large frying pan or kettle over medium heat. Add the onion, oregano and basil. Sauté them for about 1 minute, or until the onions are tender. Add the greens and sauté them until they are wilted, about 1 or 2 minutes. Swiss chard may require a few minutes longer. Turn off the heat, add the vinegar, toss and serve.

Spinach Salad with Honey Mustard Dressing

Leafy green vegetables, such as spinach, are bitter in flavor and excellent for reducing kapha. This flavorful salad should satisfy anyone's appetite. Serve with rye crackers or rice cakes.

SALAD:

1 pound (500 g) fresh spinach (washed, trimmed and chopped)
2 cups (225 g) shredded carrot
1/2 pound (250 g) fresh mushrooms, trimmed and sliced
2 cups (475 g) garbanzo beans, cooked
4 hard-boiled eggs, chopped

DRESSING:

3/4 cup (185 ml) canola oil
3 tablespoons apple cider vinegar or balsamic vinegar
3 tablespoons Dijon mustard
2 tablespoons honey
1/4 teaspoon dry mustard

To make the salad: Combine the vegetables, beans and eggs in a large bowl.

To make the dressing: Combine the remaining ingredients in a jar and shake to blend. Pour the dressing over the salad, toss and serve.

Chicken with Apple-Ginger Marinade

Apples and ginger are both good for balancing kapha. This recipe combines them with chicken to create a fruity, spicy entree. Serve with Kasha (opposite) and Steamed Broccoli (page 105).

1/2 cup (125 ml) apple juice
I clove garlic, minced, or 1/8 teaspoon garlic powder
I tablespoon peeled and minced fresh ginger or 1/4 teaspoon
   powdered ginger
I tablespoon canola oil
I pound (500 g) chicken pieces, skinned (breasts, thighs or drumsticks)
I cup (240 g) apple butter
I apple, cut into 8 wedges

To make the marinade: Combine the apple juice, garlic, ginger and oil in a large bowl or baking pan. Add the chicken to the marinade, making sure the chicken is well coated with the marinade. Cover and refrigerate for several hours or overnight.

Heat the oven to 300°F (150°C). Drain the marinade from the chicken and place the chicken in a baking pan. Spread the apple butter evenly over the chicken pieces. Place the apple wedges in the pan with the chicken. Bake, uncovered, for about 45 minutes if the chicken is on the bone, or for about 35 minutes if the chicken is boneless.

Kasha

Kasha, or roasted buckwheat, is a delicious grain product that makes a good substitute for rice.

2 cups (500 ml) low-sodium broth (chicken or vegetable)
2 tablespoons ghee or butter
$1/8$ teaspoon salt
$1/8$ teaspoon freshly ground black pepper
I egg
I cup (165 g) kasha, uncooked

In a saucepan, heat the broth, ghee or butter, salt and pepper until the mixture boils. Remove the pan from the heat and set it aside.

In a bowl, lightly beat the egg with a fork. Add the kasha to the bowl and stir it until the kernels are coated with egg. In a medium skillet or saucepan, add the egg-coated kasha. Cook the kasha over high heat for 2 or 3 minutes, stirring constantly, until the egg has dried and the kernels are separated. Reduce the heat to low.

Stir in the boiled liquid. Cover the pan and simmer for 7 to 10 minutes, until the kasha is tender and the liquid is absorbed.

Aussie Chicken

This recipe was given to me by a friend from Australia, hence the name "Aussie" chicken. This chicken has a great herbal flavor. It can be barbecued over hot coals or broiled in the oven. Serve with rye rolls and Steamed Cabbage (opposite).

1/2 cup (75 g) chopped onion
I cup (250 ml) lowfat Italian salad dressing
2 tablespoons low-sodium soy sauce
3 tablespoons chopped fresh basil or I tablespoon dried basil
I tablespoon snipped fresh rosemary or I teaspoon dried rosemary
1/2 teaspoon dried thyme
I pound (500 g) chicken pieces, skinned (breasts, thighs or drumsticks)

To make the marinade: Combine the onion, salad dressing, soy sauce, basil, rosemary and thyme in a large bowl or baking pan. Add the chicken to the marinade, making sure the chicken is well-coated. Cover and refrigerate the chicken for several hours or overnight. Drain off most of the marinade before cooking, reserving about 1/2 cup (125 ml) of the marinade.

Preheat the broiler. Place the chicken pieces on the broiler pan. Place the pan 5 inches beneath the broiling element and cook for about 6 minutes. Turn the chicken over, brush with a little reserved marinade, and cook for another 6 minutes.

Steamed Cabbage

1 small head cabbage, rinsed

Slice the cabbage into 4 wedges. Cut the hard core from each wedge. Boil 2 cups (500 ml) of water in a large saucepan or kettle. Drop the cabbage wedges into the boiling water. Cover the pan and steam the cabbage for about 10 minutes over medium heat. Drain well and serve with a little ghee or butter, if desired.

Turkey Loaf

This meat loaf recipe combines ground turkey with herbs and minced vegetables. A little orange juice adds some zip. Serve with baked potato, cranberry sauce and Succotash (page 93).

2 eggs, beaten
6 fresh medium-sized mushrooms, minced, or I small can (2 oz/60 g)
   mushroom pieces, minced
$^1/_2$ cup (55 g) shredded carrot
$^1/_4$ cup (65 ml) orange juice
$^1/_2$ cup (45 g) breadcrumbs
I tablespoon oat bran
$^1/_8$ teaspoon dried thyme
$^1/_8$ teaspoon dried marjoram, savory or sage
2 tablespoons minced fresh parsley or I teaspoon dried parsley
$^1/_4$ teaspoon freshly ground black pepper
I pound (500 g) ground turkey or ground chicken

Preheat the oven to 350°F (175°C). In a large bowl, combine the eggs, mushrooms, carrot, orange juice, breadcrumbs, oat bran, thyme, marjoram, parsley and pepper. Add the turkey and mix well. Press the mixture evenly into a 9-inch (23-cm) pie pan or a loaf pan. Bake it for 35 minutes. Remove the pan from the oven and drain off the fat. Let the loaf stand for about 10 minutes before serving.

VARIATION: *Serve sliced, cold turkey loaf on a sandwich. Go easy on the mayonnaise, or use the lowfat variety, because it tends to increase kapha. A little ketchup can substitute for the mayonnaise. I like sliced turkey loaf on rye bread with a thin layer of cranberry sauce.*

Turkey and Lentil Stew

If you like stews, you'll love this version. It's hearty, yet low in calories. Serve with rye bread or Irish Soda Bread (page 142).

1 tablespoon canola oil
1 pound (500 g) turkey breast, boned and skinned, cut into 1-inch (2.5-cm)
   cubes
¹/₄ cup (35 g) chopped onion
¹/₂ cup (50 g) chopped carrot
¹/₄ cup (25 g) chopped celery
1 clove garlic, minced
2 cups (500 ml) low-sodium broth (chicken or vegetable)
¹/₂ cup (100 g) uncooked lentils
1 can (15 oz/475 g) pureed tomatoes
1 bay leaf
1 tablespoon chopped fresh herbs or 1 teaspoon dried herbs
   (such as rosemary, marjoram, savory or thyme)

In a soup kettle or large Dutch oven, heat the oil over medium heat. Add the turkey cubes and sauté them on all sides until they are lightly browned, about 2 minutes. Remove the turkey from the pot and set it aside. Add the onion, carrot, celery, garlic and 2 tablespoons of the broth to the pot. Sauté this for about 2 minutes. Stir in the lentils and tomatoes. Then stir in the turkey cubes, bay leaf, herbs and the remaining broth. Simmer over medium-low heat for 45 minutes. Remove the bay leaf before serving.

Chicken Soup

After serving a whole roast chicken or turkey, this is a very tasty way
to make use of the carcass. This hearty soup is an age-old remedy for
the common cold, a classic kapha condition. The recipe makes about
12 servings, and if you can't eat it within a few days, it freezes very
well. Serve with rye bread or Irish Soda Bread (page 142).

1 large chicken carcass or small turkey carcass
4 small potatoes, cut into 1-inch (2.5-cm) cubes
1 large turnip, cut into 1-inch (2.5-cm) cubes
4 carrots, sliced in rounds
2 stalks celery (with leaves), chopped
1 large onion, chopped
1 small head of cabbage, cored and shredded
1 can (15 oz/475 g) chopped or puréed tomatoes
1/2 cup (100 g) barley, uncooked
1 tablespoon Worcestershire sauce
1 bay leaf
1 teaspoon dried parsley
1 teaspoon dried basil
1/4 teaspoon dried marjoram, savory or sage
1/8 teaspoon dried thyme
1/4 teaspoon freshly ground black pepper

Place the carcass in a large pot or kettle. Cover it with water and
bring it to a boil. Cover the pot, reduce the heat to low and simmer
for 1 hour. Remove the carcass from the broth. Let both carcass and
broth cool for about 15 minutes. Remove the meat from the bones
and discard the bones.

Return the meat to the broth and add the potatoes, turnip, carrots,
celery, onion, cabbage, tomatoes, barley, Worcestershire sauce, bay
leaf, parsley, basil, marjoram, thyme and pepper. Simmer the soup for
about 1 hour. Remove the bay leaf before serving.

Chili

This is a warm and satisfying meal. If you like it really spicy, add more chili powder or some dried red pepper flakes. Vegetarians can eliminate the ground turkey. Serve with Buttermilk Cornbread (page 138).

1 tablespoon ghee or canola oil
1/2 cup (75 g) chopped onion
1/2 cup (85 g) chopped green bell pepper
1/2 pound (250 g) ground turkey or chicken
2 cups (500 g) beans, cooked (such as red beans, chili beans, pinto
  beans or kidney beans)
2 large tomatoes, chopped, or 1 can (15 oz/475 g) chopped tomatoes
1 tablespoon chili powder
1/4 teaspoon garlic powder

Heat the ghee or oil over medium heat in a large frying pan. Add the onion and peppers. Sauté them for about 1 minute, or until they are tender. Stir in the ground turkey and brown it for about 3 minutes, stirring often. Add the beans, tomatoes, chili powder and garlic powder. Mix well. Bring the mixture to a boil and then reduce the heat and simmer for about 10 minutes.

Buttermilk Cornbread

1 1/2 cups (375 ml) buttermilk
2 eggs
1/4 cup (50 g) sugar
1/2 teaspoon salt
1/2 teaspoon baking soda
1 1/2 cups (200 g) corn meal
1/2 cup (50 g) all-purpose flour
1/4 cup (65 ml) melted ghee or butter

Preheat the oven to 425°F (220°C). In a large bowl, beat together the buttermilk, eggs, sugar, salt and baking soda. Stir in the corn meal and flour. Add the melted ghee or butter and mix well. Pour the batter into a greased 8-inch (20-cm)-square baking pan. Bake for 30 minutes.

Taco Salad

Spicy dressing is what makes this taco salad a real favorite in my household. I recommend using Romaine lettuce because it contains more nutrients than other varieties of lettuce. Traditionally, taco salad contains shredded cheese. Skip the cheese when balancing kapha. Serve with Corn on the Cob (page 47).

I cup (125 g) chopped cooked chicken
I cup (250 g) beans, cooked (pinto or garbanzo beans)
I head lettuce, sliced into very thin shreds
2 large or 4 small tomatoes, chopped or cut into wedges
¹/2 pound (250 g) summer squash, chopped
2 tablespoons minced scallions
3 tablespoons chopped fresh coriander leaves (cilantro)
2 tablespoons canola oil
2 tablespoons red wine vinegar
2 tablespoons salsa
2 tablespoons water
¹/2 teaspoon chili powder
¹/2 teaspoon curry powder
¹/8 teaspoon garlic powder
2 cups (75 g) tortilla chips, broken into small pieces (preferably the
  unsalted or low-salt variety)

Toss together the chicken, beans, lettuce, tomatoes, squash, scallions and fresh coriander in a large bowl.

To make the dressing: Combine the remaining ingredients in a jar (except the chips). Cover, shake well and pour over the salad. Sprinkle on the chips before serving.

Barley Pilaf

Barley, unlike wheat, is a relatively dry grain that is good for reducing kapha. This simple recipe is a wonderful grain dish to serve with a meal of poultry and vegetables, or with the vegetables alone. I recommend serving it with Steamed Brussels Sprouts (opposite).

I tablespoon canola oil
¹/₂ cup (75 g) chopped onion
¹/₂ cup (55 g) shredded carrot
I cup (200 g) uncooked pearl barley
2 cups (500 ml) low-sodium broth (chicken or vegetable)

In a medium frying pan or saucepan, heat the oil over medium heat. Add the onion and carrot and sauté for 3 minutes. Rinse and drain the barley, then sauté with the onion and carrot for 1 additional minute. Add the broth, stir and bring the mixture to a boil. Cover and cook over medium-low heat for 30 minutes.

Steamed Brussels Sprouts

I pound (500 g) Brussels sprouts
2 tablespoons ghee or butter, melted
2 teaspoons fresh lemon juice or apple cider vinegar

Rinse the sprouts and cut off the tough ends. Bring 2 cups of water
to a boil. Drop the sprouts into the boiling water. Cover the pan.
Steam over medium heat for about 10 minutes. Drain them well. Mix
the ghee or butter with the lemon juice or vinegar in a small bowl.
Drizzle this mixture over the sprouts before serving.

Irish Soda Bread

Raisins and caraway seeds make this very easy bread recipe a tasty treat. Half of the flour used in this version of soda bread is barley flour. This will make the bread a little drier, thereby helping to balance kapha. Serve with soups, such as Chicken Soup (page 136), or salads, such as Spinach Salad with Honey Mustard Dressing (page 129).

1 1/2 cups (150 g) all-purpose flour
1 1/2 cups (150 g) barley flour
2 teaspoons baking powder
1 teaspoon baking soda
1 teaspoon salt
1 tablespoon caraway seeds
1 cup (150 g) raisins or currants
1 1/4 cups (300 ml) buttermilk
2 tablespoons canola oil

Preheat the oven to 375°F (190°C). In a large mixing bowl, stir together the two flours, baking powder, baking soda, salt and caraway seeds. Stir in the raisins. In a small bowl, mix together the buttermilk and oil. Stir the buttermilk mixture into the flour mixture to make a soft dough. Turn the dough onto a lightly floured board or counter and gently knead it for 1 minute. Flatten the dough until it is about 8 inches (20 cm) in diameter. Place the flattened dough on a greased cookie sheet or in a greased 8-inch (20-cm)-round baking pan. Cut a few shallow slits in the top of the dough. Bake for about 45 minutes, until the top is golden-brown.

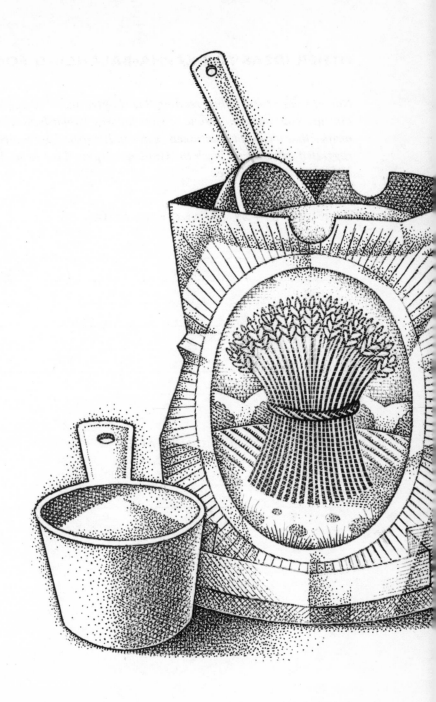

OTHER IDEAS FOR KAPHA-BALANCING FOODS

Now it's your turn! While reading this chapter on balancing kapha, I'm sure you thought of some of your favorite kapha-balancing recipes that were not mentioned. You can list them here under the suggested categories. Check the Guidelines (page 116) to see if any adjustments are required.

MAIN DISHES FOR BALANCING KAPHA:

_____

_____

_____

_____

_____

_____

_____

DESSERTS FOR BALANCING KAPHA:

_____

_____

_____

SNACKS FOR BALANCING KAPHA:

_____

_____

_____

BEVERAGES FOR BALANCING KAPHA:

_____

_____

_____

BREAKFASTS FOR BALANCING KAPHA:

_____

_____

_____

DINING OUT

These days, not many people eat all their meals at home. Most of us visit a restaurant or two during the course of a week. How do we follow Ayurvedic guidelines when making a restaurant menu selection? It's really not as difficult as it might seem. Keep in mind the types of foods that are recommended for reducing the dosha you're trying to balance. Then find these foods on the restaurant's menu. If they don't appear on the menu, go to a restaurant more likely to serve the foods you want. The following is a summary of foods to look for when balancing each dosha, and a list of the restaurants likely to serve those foods.

VATA

To balance vata, eat rich, warm, well-cooked foods. Emphasize naturally sweet, salty and sour foods. Nonvegetarians can eat poultry and seafood. Appropriate restaurants include:

- Asian
- Italian
- Pizza
- Seafood
- Mexican
- Fast food (for an occasional chicken or fish sandwich)
- Pancake
- French
- Vegetarian

PITTA

To balance pitta, look for light, cooling foods. Dry, raw foods such as salads are good. Emphasize foods that are naturally sweet, bitter and astringent. Nonvegetarians can eat poultry and small amounts of shrimp. Appropriate restaurants include:

- Salad bars
- Sandwich shops
- Oriental (avoid the spicy selections)
- French (light selections)
- Fast food (salads)
- Vegetarian

KAPHA

To balance kapha, eat mostly warm foods. Keep meals light. Emphasize foods that are spicy, bitter and astringent in flavor. Nonvegetarians can eat poultry. Appropriate restaurants include:

- Asian (particularly the spicy selections)
- East Indian
- Mexican (avoid cheese and sour cream)
- Middle Eastern
- Barbecued chicken
- Vegetarian

RESOURCES

BOOKS ABOUT AYURVEDA

Chopra, Deepak. *Perfect Health: The Complete Mind/Body Guide*. New York, NY: Harmony Books, 1991. A personal manual on using the principles of Ayurveda to achieve perfect health. Part I defines "perfect health" and explains its relationship to the doshas. Part II describes basic treatments and therapies. Part III is a practical guide to daily routine, with an excellent chapter on diet.

Frawley, David. *Ayurvedic Healing: A Comprehensive Guide*. Salt Lake City, UT: Passage Press, 1989. An excellent reference book on Ayurveda. Basic Ayurvedic principles are covered in Part I. Part II discusses treatments for common diseases. Part III presents information on Ayurvedic herbs, tonics and other classic remedies.

Lad, Vasant. *Ayurveda, The Science of Self-Healing: A Practical Guide*. Santa Fe, NM: Lotus Press, 1985. An excellent introduction and personal guidebook to Ayurveda. One chapter describes a wide array of commonly available natural substances that can be used as herbal treatments.

—.*The Complete Book of Ayurvedic Home Remedies*. New York, NY: Three Rivers Press, 1998. Following a very clear introduction and a self-test for determining your constitution in Part I, Part II provides techniques for cleansing the body, suggestions for your daily routine, breathing techniques, meditation techniques and dietary guidelines. Part III is the real gem of this book—a section on illnesses and Ayurvedic remedies from "A to Z."

Reddy, Kumuda, and Stan Kendz. *Forever Healthy: Introduction to Maharishi Ayur-Veda Health Care*. Rochester, NY: Samhita Enterprises, 1997. This book describes all of the components of the Maharishi Ayur-Veda system of natural health care. The Maharishi Ayur-Veda Program offers various therapies including meditation, pulse diagnosis, herbal formulas and seasonal rejuvenation treatments. The publisher of this book, Samhita Enterprises, has an Internet site containing information on Ayurveda. The web page address is: http://www.samhita.com.

Shanbhag, Vivek. *A Beginner's Introduction to Ayurvedic Medicine*. New Canaan, CT: Keats Publishing, Inc., 1994. This short guidebook provides a succinct introduction to Ayurveda. Included is a self-test to determine Ayurvedic constitution and a list of foods that help balance each dosha.

Svoboda, Robert E. *Prakruti: Your Ayurvedic Constitution*. Albuquerque, NM: Geocom Limited, 1989. An invaluable book for truly understanding human Ayurvedic constitutional types. Contains helpful chapters on food and nutrition.

AYURVEDIC COOKBOOKS

Banchek, Linda. *The AyurVeda Cookbook: Cooking for Life*. Fairfield, IA: Orchids & Herbs Press, 1990. Contains background information about Ayurveda and food. The wide variety of vegetarian recipes includes beverages, appetizers, salads, dressings and sauces, condiments, breads, soups, main dishes and desserts. An appendix contains a list of foods showing the effect each has on the doshas.

Johari, Harish. *The Healing Cuisine: India's Art of Ayurvedic Cooking*. Rochester, VT: Healing Arts Press, 1994. Contains classic Indian-style vegetarian recipes that follow Ayurvedic principles. The introductory section explains Ayurvedic principles and describes the properties of many main ingredients. Recipe categories include snacks, dals, rice dishes, vegetable dishes, paneer dishes, yogurt dishes, salads, condiments, breads, desserts and beverages.

Morningstar, Amadea, and Urmila Desai. *The Ayurvedic Cookbook: A Personalized Guide to Good Nutrition and Health*. Santa Fe, NM: Lotus Press, 1990. Begins with an introduction to Ayurveda, which contains a self-test on discovering your constitution. Includes sample daily menus for vata, pitta and kapha. The vegetarian recipes include main dishes, vegetables, condiments, desserts, beverages and breakfasts. An appendix contains a list of foods to increase or decrease for balancing each dosha.

Tiwari, Maya. *Ayurveda, A Life of Balance: The Complete Guide to Ayurvedic Nutrition and Body Types with Recipes*. Rochester, VT: Healing Arts Press, 1995. Provides a very thorough explanation of the Ayurvedic body types (constitutions) from both a physical and mental perspective. Lists foods that balance each body type. The second half of the book contains vegetarian recipes, each with adaptations for different body types.

AYURVEDIC ORGANIZATIONS

There are many Ayurvedic health centers and clinics in the United States. The following three national organizations were chosen because they offer a wide range of services, including herbal products, treatments and courses on Ayurveda.

The Ayurveda Institute, 11311 Menaul Blvd. NE, Albuquerque, NM 87192-1445. Phone number: 505/291-9698. Web: http://www.ayurveda.com

The Chopra Center for Well-Being, 2013 Costa del Mar Road, Carlsbad, CA 92009. Toll-free phone number: 888/424-6772. Web: http://www.chopra.com

Maharishi Ayurveda Products, 1068 Elkton Drive, Colorado Springs, CO 80907. Toll-free phone number: 800/255-8332. Web: http://www.mapi.com

RECIPE INDEX